NURSING MANAGEMENT

Concepts, Functions, Techniques and Skills

Joan M. Ganong, R. N. , M. S.

and

Warren L. Ganong, C. M. C.

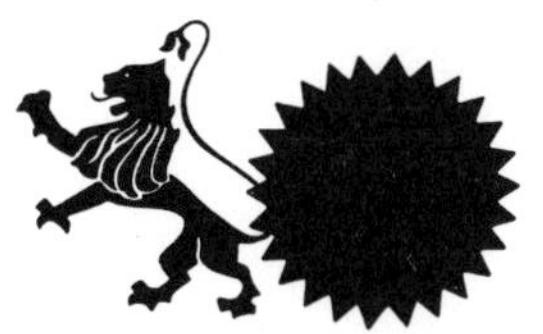

Aspen Systems Corporation
Germantown, Maryland
1976

Copyright © 1976 by Aspen Systems Corporation

Library of Congress Catalog Card Number: 76-29787
ISBN: 0-912862-30-0

Printed in the United States of America.
2 3 4 5

Table of Contents

List of Tables and Figures

Preface

This is a book not only for nurse managers but for all nurses, including
students of nursing, since all nurses use the management process in
their work. Often they use it not recognizing it by that name. Every
nurse learns and uses—or is expected to use—the four steps of the
nursing process: assessing, planning, implementing and evaluating.
The nursing process model is based upon the same model as the
management process of planning, doing and controlling.

Our purpose is to provide a practical, easy-to-use guide to the
understanding and implementation of management concepts, functions, techniques and skills as they apply in healthcare agencies. Thus
the book will be helpful to nurse managers at all levels of responsibility in hospitals, nursing homes, public health agencies, mental health
clinics, schools of nursing and related facilities providing all types of
acute, short-term, extended, home, in- and outpatient healthcare services and education. Nurses who have their own independent practices
can benefit from this book as fully as those in the customary agencies.
Our theme is effective management of patient care as provided by
nurses, in whatever setting, to the healthcare consumer (i.e. the pa-
tient/client/person seeking assistance as an individual or as a member
of a group). We elaborate on this theme through a continuing emphasis
on the management process as carried out by nurses who understand
and use the management functions, techniques and skills. We build
upon proven concepts and practices of modern management as they
are being successfully applied by nurses in an ever growing number of
healthcare agencies. Our focus is always on the management of pa-
tient/client care and services—with all of the implications suggested
by that phrase. (Throughout the book we use "patient" to designate
the person who is the recipient of services, recognizing that other
terms are more appropriate in particular settings.) Whenever we use
the phrase "management of patient care," we do so only within the
broad meaning which includes the patient's direct involvement in the

patient care process (or, when necessary, with the involvement of the patient's family and/or significant others).

Our psychological orientation is more humanistic than behavioral, more Maslovian than Freudian or Skinnerian. We subscribe to the third-force concepts of Abraham Maslow. This is apparent throughout our professional work and throughout this book. We believe that helping others to meet their own needs is the most potent motivational force available to managers and nurses. We strive to strike an appropriate balance in the use of the technical mode and the human mode in the practice of management. This kind of goal-oriented management seeks to create a working environment in which all employees are encouraged to participate to the maximum extent possible in decisions affecting them and their work.

The rights movement affects us all. All of us are caught up in the thrust toward a better way of recognizing human rights — or more accurately, of helping others to recognize their right, their natural human drive, to strive toward a satisfaction of their human needs. We encourage nurse managers to adopt this realistic view of rights — be they patients' rights, employee rights, women's rights, minority rights, managers' rights, doctors' rights, or nurses' rights. This will continue as a significant challenge to each of us.*

The greatest demand for numbers of nurse managers is within institutional settings. Thus, many of our examples are drawn from hospitals and related types of healthcare agencies. At the same time, all of the materials included herein have direct application in other types of settings such as community mental health centers, public health departments and independent nursing practice. The problem-oriented nursing system, the nursing process, performance evaluation, patient teaching, nursing by objectives, budgetary planning and control, motivation and leadership — these and other essentials in the effective delivery of patient care services are treated consistently as interrelated components of a humanistically oriented management process.

Our use of the term "nurse manager" rather than "administrator" is deliberate. The term "manager" is an all-inclusive term and includes any person whose title is administrator or director. By definition, an administrator is one who performs management functions at the executive level. A manager is one who manages others and who provides leadership for individual and group activity. (See the Glossary for definitions of management terms used throughout this book.)

---

*For some startling documentation, see Robert W. Cunningham, Jr., "The Shroud of Silence is Wearing Thin," *Modern Healthcare* 22 (January 1976), p10.

In summary, our purposes in this book are to:

1. Set forth a philosophy of nursing management that embraces enunciated value concepts, the importance of each individual as part of the work group, goal-oriented management practices, the time-tested motivational theory of Abraham Maslow, and the precepts of humanistic psychology that both recognize and transcend individual differences.

2. Contribute toward the understanding and use of modern management concepts in nursing practice and education.

3. Present problem-oriented nursing as a system for managing patient care, and describe the organizational structure required to support it.

4. Explain the management functions, techniques, and skills that are necessary to implement the foregoing.

5. Provide specific guidance in the use of the management process for the benefit of patients, staff, employees, and the community at large.

6. Emphasize the financial impact of the nurse manager's performance, and how to achieve a necessary balance between patient care goals and the realities of budgetary planning and control.

This book is organized into four parts: Part I provides an overview of the workworld of the nurse manager. Each individual manager is viewed as the center of his/her working environment. Personal attributes and environmental factors are described that influence each person's performance as nurse, as manager, and as a professional in a helping relationship to others. The three major areas of responsibility of the nurse manager are described as patient care management (the clinical aspects), operational management (the business-related aspects), and human resources management (the personnel and staff development aspects.)

The understanding of and ability to use management concepts, functions, techniques and skills are seen as necessary supportive elements to permit adequate performance of nurse manager responsibilities. Also stressed are the requirements of a suitable organizational structure with adequate policies and practices, not only in nursing but throughout the agency as a whole.

Parts II, III, and IV deal with each of the three major areas of the nurse manager's responsibility. Part II presents the Problem-Oriented Nursing System (PONS) as the process model for patient care management. Five essential components of PONS are described. These are the foundation (the principles of nursing practice), the nursing process, the problem-oriented nursing record (PONR), nursing audit, and education (for patients and staff).

Part III deals with operational management. Specific management techniques are explained, with emphasis on their importance in achieving patient care goals. The selected techniques, presented in sufficient detail to serve as a guide to their implementation, are management by objectives, results-oriented performance evaluation, nursing audit and annual budgetary planning and control.

Part IV deals with human resources management. Particular attention is given to motivation, employee relations, patient and staff education, and the wide-track careers concept in nursing.

The history of nursing has been exciting and meaningful. It is an integral part of our country's striving. The new nurse managers, poised now at the threshold of the nation's third century, will exert an increasingly potent force on the future of us all. We wish them well.

Chapel Hill, North Carolina   Joan and Warren Ganong
November 1976

Acknowledgments

Books represent people—first of all, their authors, but also significant others. We are keenly aware of the impact on us of many persons whose lives and work have touched ours and whom we recognize as having contributed much to us and, hence, to this book. Among these are Dr. Margaret E. Courtney of Johns Hopkins University and Hospital; Dr. Florence M. Gipe, Dean Emeritus of the School of Nursing at the University of Maryland; Doris E. Gosnell, Director of Nursing for Staff Development, Aultman Hospital, Canton, Ohio; Asa S. Knowles, Chancellor of Northeastern University; Dr. Ruth P. Kuehn, Dean Emeritus of the School of Nursing, University of Pittsburgh; the late Dr. Abraham H. Maslow, Chairman of the Department of Psychology at Brandeis University; Edward H. Noroian, Vice President, Temple University Hospital; Gearlean M. Slack, formerly Director of Continuing Education, School of Nursing at West Virginia University; and John M. Watkins, Publisher, Contemporary Publishing, Inc.

We offer sincere thanks to the wide spectrum of authors and publishers whose works are continuing sources of inspiration and help, many of whom are noted herein. A special word of appreciation is due to our consulting and workshop clients whose productive creativity in achieving on-the-job implementation results has been so meaningful and satisfying—to us, to them, and to their patients.

We appreciate the efforts and ready cooperation, patience, and skill of Barbara Hoecke and Anita Marten of our own staff in producing the manuscript. We are proud to have such fine people helping us speak to you through this book.

Part I

Workworld of the Nurse Manager

Chapter 1
The Nurse in the Organization

One of the reasons for studying nursing is to become a professional helper. Nurses learn how to provide skilled help to other persons with healthcare needs. The student of nursing typically learns to visualize the nursing role as a one-to-one relationship between the individual as nurse and another individual as patient. And so it may be. But more often than not the graduate nurse begins to practice nursing as a member of a complex organization—a healthcare agency made up of groups of individuals with varied competencies who provide necessary services for the patients or clients being served.

You undoubtedly first began to realize the need for finding your place in a healthcare organizational hierarchy as a student. You learned to understand your role within the formal organizational structure of a nursing department, and became familiar with the complexities of the interrelationships among departments, professional disciplines, patients, employee groups and administration. You may have begun to wonder then, or later, how you could achieve the type of nurse-patient relationship once visualized. As a student you learned that your function was to become well acquainted with the needs and problems of each individual patient and then to use your knowledge and skills to help meet those patient needs in a personal way. Instead, as a staff nurse you were assigned a workload of tasks, procedures and routines for a group of patients being served en masse by a variety of members of the patient care team. You observed too that those nurses who progressed to higher-level nursing positions spent less and less time in individual patient care and learned that to progress in your profession and earn higher monetary rewards you would have to accept responsibility for others as a head nurse or supervisor.

For years this has been true and is still true in many organizations. Yet today in most areas of the healthcare industry, nurses are finding that they can make progress professionally and financially without moving into the ranks of management. Job opportunities and earnings on the clinical track parallel those on the management track. Job titles such as clinical specialist, nurse clinician, primary nurse, nurse practitioner and nursing consultant are providing new advancement opportunities.

This trend is a healthy one and has opened up career opportunities heretofore unavailable to nurses. Yet there is a sometimes unrecognized aspect of what has been happening. The entire concept of the nurse manager function has been changing. The role that was once seen as a supervisory link in a traditional authoritarian chain-of- command hierarchy has been changing toward the concept of a nurse manager who performs as a true facilitator-coordinator-leader. This is a potent change and one which we seek to encourage. It is based upon the weight of experience as well as the findings of the behavioral sciences.

Another change is also having an impact on nursing. This is the trend toward greater accountability by individual nurse practitioners in every work setting. While it has always been true that all professional persons have been accountable for their actions, there is now a far greater stress than ever before upon clearly defined standards of practice and the auditing of results. This is another aspect of the rights movement. One by-product is a clear recognition that the practice of enlightened management is vital. In fact, it is critical to the future of nursing in the world of healthcare. The nurse as clinician and the nurse as manager must understand and practice—thoughtfully and deliberately—the necessary management functions, techniques and skills to carry out their performance responsibilities. Professional nurses, by virtue of being licensed to practice, have always been expected to assume responsibility for supervising the work of others in lower job categories. From this point of view nurses always have had the responsibility of managerial leadership and its attendant accountability. But in today's workworld the professional nurse has both expanded opportunities and more clearly defined responsibilities to apply management principles and practices, whether they choose the clinical, education or management track as a career plan. In fact, more and more nurses find it beneficial to switch back and forth among these three tracks. In doing so they enhance their ability to use their management knowledge and skills. Thus the term "nurse manager" can be used with either of two different emphases—"*nurse* manager" or "nurse *manager.*"

This dual role of nurse and manager applies at every job level in nursing. Whether as staff nurse, head nurse or administrator, the professional nurse necessarily is both nurse and manager with the emphasis shifting according to need. As *nurse* manager, the emphasis is upon the nurse as clinician practicing one's own professional nursing skills. This may be done simply as another RN member of the patient care staff on a unit, with only nominal responsibility for the work performed by nonnurses within the group. (Here the nurse is managing as a professional helper for one's own patients.) Or the nurse-as-clinician may be serving as a primary nurse or team leader with a more apparent leadership role vis-a-vis the other members of the immediate patient care staff. Or the nurse may be acting as a charge nurse or assistant head nurse with temporary shift responsibility for the management of patient care provided by the unit personnel available for that shift—often a highly mobile group of persons in today's hospital environment. In each of these situations the emphasis tends to be on the nurse-as-clinician providing personal patient care, albeit with a group of helpers to assist with the patient care services. Minimal attention is focused on the managerial components of these roles, except as the individual nurse recognizes his/her professional responsibility for patient care management. The personnel management responsibility, even if recognized, often cannot be assumed effectively. The reasons for this are many and include the nature of the nurse's education, the confusion as to who is really in charge of the unit personnel at any given time, and the inability of nursing administration to establish an effective, decentralized organizational structure appropriate for a modern healthcare agency.

The nurse *manager* role, in contrast, places the emphasis upon the nurse as a professional manager. The nursing knowledge, skills and philosophy are still essential. The clinical skills will be practiced less and less as the nurse progresses to the higher level of management positions, but the other components of being a nurse will continue to be a requirement. One of the reasons for this is the need for credibility and acceptance of persons in the top leadership positions of the key department in any agency devoted to helping patients meet their healthcare needs. Nursing is, and will remain for the foreseeable future, the key department in such agencies. It is the department that provides patient care services twenty-four hours a day, seven days a week throughout the year. It is the department that spends upwards of forty percent of the operating budget of a typical hospital. It has more people on the payroll than any other department. Clearly, the nurses in charge must be competent managers. This requirement applies at all levels beginning with the assistant head nurses and charge nurses.

In view of the foregoing and recognizing the dual clinical/managerial roles of any professional nurse, the contents of this book are intended primarily to assist the nurse *manager* in the role of charge nurse, head nurse, supervisor, coordinator, assistant director, associate director, director of nursing service, director of nursing, vice president for patient care services, chief nurse, college dean, director of nursing education, coordinator of healthcare occupations, inservice education director, director of continuing education, staff development director and so on. Titles abound. Yet they reflect common management components. Our focus is on these components.

YOUR WORKWORLD BEGINS WITH YOU

You are, quite literally, the center of your workworld. You are unique. Thus your job situation is unique. Regardless of your title, job or performance description, and the nature of the supervision you receive, your workworld is more you than anything else. You have more influence on your job situation, more responsibility and more authority to act than you may realize or utilize. This is a fact often overlooked. Nurses in almost every position are known to complain, "If only I had the authority to go with my responsibility!" Or "I could be much more effective if only I didn't have to get an O.K. on everything from my boss." And "Why can't we make more of our own decisions right here on our own unit?"

Yet the managers of these same nurses have complaints of their own. They often say, "If only my people would show some initiative! Why won't they make a decision on their own? They don't have to check with me all the time." Such comments reflect organizational relationships that are all too common. When such ambiguity about role relationships is allowed to continue, the fault lies with both parties—the superior and the subordinate. The manager, recognizing a situation in which subordinates are not willing to make decisions that are within the scope of their responsibility and authority, should take the necessary steps to clarify whatever misunderstandings exist. Sometimes the problem is simply a matter of one person misunderstanding the expectations of the other. Frank discussion can clear the air. Other times the problem involves the complications and nuances of decision making that are in gray areas of role responsibility and authority. The manager's dictum of "When in doubt, check with me," is not adequate except in cases of long-standing relationships. It too easily becomes a crutch for the unsure or indecisive subordinate.

A useful tool that the manager can use in discussions with subordinates is a Decision Worksheet to outline the degrees of responsibility and authority. On one side list typical situations and problems found in the nursing situation and on the other a range of action possibilities of which one could be checked off as applicable to the situation. Five action possibilities, coded by letters, are: (A) I act on my own initiative. No need to inform others of my action. (B) I take action, and inform my boss (and possibly others) afterward. (C) I consult my boss in advance and say what I expect to do. (D) I recommend action to be carried out by my boss (or others). (E) I turn over the problem to my boss (or others) with no recommendation for action. The use of this form will help to explore and resolve areas of uncertainty in the minds of the manager and the subordinates.

The person in the subordinate position has responsibility too for initiating action to clarify questions about decision-making authority. Once familiar with the Decision Worksheet, the subordinate can fill it in for a range of typical situations and problems.

For example, Peggy Ansel (a head nurse) might select the following problems and indicate the level of action responsibility she believes her own nurse manager expects of her.

PROBLEM	A	B	C	D	E
1. Nurse does not update care plans daily	X				
2. Doctor wants a new set up for stocking treatment cart			X		
3. Nurse aide claims discrimination in work assignments		X			
4. Patient says watch was stolen	X				
5. My neighbor reports that our housekeepers are taking steps to join a union					X
6. Night supervisor provides inadequate patient care support on my unit				X	
7. Unit secretary needs to be replaced			X		

Having completed this listing, Peggy then requests an opportunity to sit down with her own manager to see if they are in agreement. Open discussion will resolve any differences. Follow-through discussions will be required to explore fully the variety of questions that may arise regarding each other's responsibility and accountability.

Another recourse for the subordinate is to "see what you can get away with." This is suggested in the positive, constructive sense of testing how far you can go in making your own decisions—by making them (within the commonsense dictates of policies, practice, and your inclination for taking risks). Decision making involves taking calculated risks. No manager can be sure of making safe decisions all of the time. As a professional, you will learn quickly through this testing approach the degree of appropriate risks you can assume in your decision making within your organization. Most nurse managers can "get away with" more than they realize—by taking on the responsibility and authority expected of them by a competent leader/facilitator.

Remember also another maxim: Never let your boss be surprised. This applies especially to your own actions and relationships. Your manager should not learn from other sources information that you could have provided sooner or more appropriately. Keep your communication lines open. Your use of the Decision Worksheet will assist in developing the empathy that is needed in an effective superior/subordinate relationship.

Each day when you enter your workworld you bring with you your values, your motivation, your knowledge and your skills. These comprise your apperceptive mass, the associational areas of your brain. What you do with these components of yourself each day affects you and others, including your personnel and your patients. These personal attributes comprise the first and central segment of a complete picture of your workworld.

Your values are obviously a highly important part of you and have a sometimes unrecognized influence upon your philosophy and actions as a nurse manager. The term "values" refers to your beliefs, attitudes, and principles that affect your life and work. What do you value? What do you believe in? What is most important to you? What is your attitude toward yourself and others? Is your list of values made up more of things than of people-related items? These are serious questions and deserve your best thought and response; for your values inevitably influence all that you do as a nurse and as a manager. They influence your use of your clinical skills and your managerial skills. They influence the way in which you react to change. Your values are influencing your response to this material at the present moment. Admittedly, most of your values are acquired subconsciously during your early years and remain relatively unchanged all of your life. Other values may grow or be shaped out of your later life and work experiences.

Your motivation is what causes you to do what you do, to select one course of action instead of another. Your human needs have a great influence on your motivation. One of the most useful and durable theories of human motivation is that of Abraham Maslow. Appendix I provides a personalized adaptation of this theory of motivation. It will serve you well in understanding yourself and others.

A third component of your apperceptive mass is your knowledge. It has been said that chance favors the prepared mind. This is a way of saying that you make your own luck and that there are certain requisites for experiencing personal satisfaction from your work. Adequate job knowledge, the kind of technical and managerial knowledge that gives you confidence in your own ability, is one such requisite. There can be no substitute for necessary job knowledge acquired through study and experience.

Competence involves not only knowing what to do but being able to do it well. You can perform satisfactorily as a nurse manager only when you have sufficient skills in both the technical and human modes of the nurse manager's role. These include both clinical and managerial skills. You acquire some of these skills prior to becoming a nurse manager. Other skills you develop as you work and learn.

The four personal components comprising your apperceptive mass are the sum total of all your education, training, life experience, parental influence, religion, jobs, prejudices, beliefs and so on. It is what you have to react with, the associational areas of your brain, your own privately-programmed built-in computer.

Perhaps you feel that you are locked into your apperceptive mass, into being the person you are. This seems to be true for most of us. And that is just fine. What you are today is O.K. But you are not a finished product and neither is anyone else. All of us are in the process of becoming, of continuing to find out how to use most effectively our own personal assets and abilities. With this in mind, let's continue to develop the picture of your workworld.

Your workworld may be an 850-bed acute care hospital, a 10-bed cardiac care unit, a 75-bed nursing home, or a 25,000-population community being served by your public health agency. Regardless of the size or nature of your particular setting, you have three major areas of responsibility. These are patient care management, operational management, and human resources management. Components of each of these responsibilities are summarized briefly as follows:

Patient Care Management	Operational Management	Human Resources Management
Assess problems and needs,	Budgeting,	Teaching,
Problem identification,	Controlling Expenses,	Counselling,
Planning of care,	Staffing,	Facilitating,
Providing care,	Providing supplies,	Rounds,
Teaching,	Scheduling,	Conferences,
Treatments,	Communicating,	In-service programs,
Medications,	Coordinating,	Continuing education,
Clinical conferences, and	Planning,	Bulletin boards,
Evaluating results;	Evaluating performance,	Journals,
	Meetings,	Career mobility,
	Auditing, and	Peer review, and
	Committees;	Research.

Clearly, every nurse manager by whatever title at each level within the nursing department has responsibilities in these three areas. The extent to which these responsibilities are recognized and discharged by individual nurse managers in a given health care agency is affected by three major factors. These factors are philosophy, delegation and competency.

The first factor is the philosophy and organizational concepts of the top administrator in the agency. This has to do with basic beliefs about people and the ways of securing effective performance. It involves ideas about teamwork, risk taking and support. It includes comprehending the messages of writers like Appley, Argyris, Drucker, Goble, Maslow, McGregor and Myers. Some administrators prefer to hold the reins tightly themselves and permit little or no initiative and assumption of responsibility by department heads and other supervisory management personnel. Other administrators believe that the best way for the agency to achieve its objectives is to delegate the maximum amount of authority, responsibility and accountability for results through a decentralized organization structure with adequate centralized control mechanisms. Such administrators tend to believe with Lawrence Appley that "management is guiding human and physical resources into dynamic organizational units that attain their objectives to the satisfaction of those served with a high degree of morale and sense of attainment on the part of those rendering the service."[1]

The second factor is the degree of delegation exercised by the top-level nurse manager. Even when the agency administrator believes in and achieves meaningful delegation of responsibility and authority, those at the next level of administration (such as the director of nursing) may not be able or willing to follow the example set for them. When this happens, those persons in the lower levels of management are likely to be restricted in exercising their full potential as managers.

The third factor is the personal competency and accountability of the nurse manager in the subordinate position (patient care coordinator or head nurse, for example). A vital component of competency has been identified as motive force, which is that element in the working relationship between two or more persons which determines whose plan of action is dominant. It is characterized by an ability to see the broad picture, a desire to change things and a willingness to be measured by results.[2]

While the nature of managerial performance responsibilities is similar at varying levels of an organization, the degree of responsibility varies depending upon the scope of the individual position. For example, a head nurse assumes only a small share of total managerial responsibility within nursing and does so for an individual patient care unit of limited size with an annual operating budget of perhaps $150,000 or less. A patient care coordinator responsible for a group of units has a broader managerial work load and may be responsible for a budget that is in the $300,000 to $700,000 range. The director of nursing service, with the full scope of nursing management responsibility in a hospital of 300 to 400 beds, may have a budget responsibility of somewhere between four and six million dollars, representing as much as 40% of the operating expense budget for the entire hospital. Obviously, other characteristics also distinguish the job of nursing director from that of head nurse. In developing the concept of the workworld of a nurse manager, the general components apply at all levels of managerial responsibility.

Now, a word about terminology. The professions — such as nursing, medicine, and law — have their own terminology and a need for the use of words that convey precise meanings. So does the field of management. As a professional nurse you have learned the necessity for the accurate use of technical terms. Similarly, as a professional manager, you need to be familiar with and make careful use of accurate management terms. Your accurate use of correct management terminology to say as clearly as possible what you mean will help to reduce misunderstanding and facilitate clear communications. And since "meanings are not in words—meanings are in people," successful communication requires more than your use of precise management terms. Clear communication requires the extra effort of an explanation in words appropriate to the comprehension level of the listener. The Glossary at the end of the book, together with our attempt to use the terminology consistently, are intended to contribute to your management communication efforts.

MANAGEMENT FUNCTIONS, TECHNIQUES AND SKILLS

A conceptualization of your workworld as a nurse manager can be seen as a supportive structure for you and your responsibilities. This supportive structure is made up of the management functions, techniques and skills. These components of managing are carried out not by you alone, but also by your own manager and by your own subordinates in their respective roles. All members of the management team require a clear understanding of the management functions, techniques and skills and how they are applied at the various organizational levels to secure achievement of objectives and goals. The primary focus of objectives and goals is providing the types of care and services that best meet the needs and problems of individual patients and clients. The performance of nurse managers has a critical influence on the caliber of results. We need to examine the ways in which optimum results can be obtained.

Management Functions

Management functions are the basic processes which comprise the work of the manager. These processes are identified as planning, doing and controlling, and their practicial application is the main thrust of this book.

Planning

Planning is thinking ahead, determining what shall be done. Planning is the process of establishing goals, defining problems and opportunities, setting objectives and developing strategy and tactics for action. Thus planning involves making decisions regarding such actions as establishing and clarifying organizational relationships; developing broad goals; establishing policies and considering how to implement them; mapping long-range programs and projects; setting specific objectives with target dates for completion; determining specific methods and procedures; fixing day-to-day work assignments and schedules; and estimating budgetary requirements.

Doing

Doing is the implementation phase of the manager's job. It involves carrying out the plans, working on the short-term objectives to achieve the broader purposes and goals. Included in this function are providing leadership and direction for the nursing staff; making use of the necessary leadership tools, techniques, skills and controls; assuring adequate materials, supplies and nursing staff; developing objectives and performance responsibilities with the personnel involved; defining standards of performance with personnel; arranging self-development opportunities for personnel; coordinating work activities, integrating viewpoints; building the kind of climate that encourages self-development, motivation and self-control by personnel; performing direct patient care as required; maintaining strong nurse manager/nursing staff relationships; controlling payroll costs and other expense items; and assuring that adequate records are kept to meet all patient care, administrative and legal requirements.

Controlling

Controlling is the evaluating, measuring and feedback function. Controlling provides the link between doing and replanning. Controlling assesses how well the doing achieved the objectives and goals of planning. Thus controlling provides the objective data for looking back at what has happened, and for looking ahead to what else you want to happen. In this manner, the recycling of the functions of management continues — the ongoing process of planning, doing and controlling.

The controlling function involves setting standards for evaluation purposes at carefully selected strategic control points; checking and reporting on performance compared with standards; taking corrective action as indicated; measuring performance results periodically against plans, (1) by appraising departmental and unit results against objectives, (2) by performance reviews, comparing individual results with the criteria for satisfactory performance and specific objectives. Controlling also includes interpreting results, then modifying or expanding existing plans to achieve revised objectives. The feedback aspect of controlling necessitates the use of a suitable performance evaluation procedure such as ROPEP (described in Part III) so that people know how they are doing and what changes, if any, are desirable for the future.

You will readily recognize that the management functions are not individually discrete parts of the managing process. They do not exist independently of each other. On the contrary, they are interdependent, overlapping and supportive segments of a continually recycling process. For example, the controlling function has to be planned or it will not be effective. And the measuring and evaluative aspects of controlling, to be most timely and useful, often need to occur during the doing function. A dramatic patient care illustration is the use of the cardiopulmonary resuscitation (CPR) team as an emergency patient care technique on a medical-surgical unit. Consider how the management functions are interrelated.

Controlling. The first indications (objective feedback from the patient) of a cardiac arrest by a medical-surgical patient on such a unit are usually identified by some member of the nursing staff. The staff member takes immediate action: "code blue" (or similar stat call) to secure the CPR team, and immediate emergency measures within the skills and responsibility of the staff member. This is doing in accordance with plan.

Doing. The feedback and evaluative signs which triggered the CPR procedure (observed as part of the controlling function) occurred during the doing function of managing the nursing care of a particular group of patients. (How soon after the patient first showed cardiac arrest symptoms were those symptoms recognized by the nursing staff? Could they have been recognized sooner? How well did the response occur? Was it effective for the patient?) The CPR procedure itself is a doing function, and must be well managed. It obviously requires meticulous planning (the advance selection and training of the CPR team members, the purchase and maintenance of equipment), prompt response and fast teamwork under skilled leadership when a call occurs, instantaneous feedback and response (controlling while doing) during the crisis, and a sense of organized, well-managed effort throughout.

Planning. Several references to planning have been identified in the controlling and doing as described above. The entire CPR procedure, of course, is a masterpiece of management—from conceptualization and planning through implementation and evaluation. The procedure brings into action the coordinated efforts of an interdisciplinary team of members who understand and are skilled in their roles, and who are led by a prepared leader—a model of management in the full sense of purposeful human activity to carry out the necessary functions, techniques and procedures with appropriate skill and dispatch.

Giving a separate identity (the functions of planning, doing and controlling) to the major segments of the managing process helps in conceptualizing what management is all about, and assists in differentiating the functions of management from the skills and techniques used by managers.

Management Techniques and Skills

As part of your personal supporting structure for carrying out your performance responsibilities, the management functions are of central importance. The other two parts of your supporting structure are identified as management techniques and management skills. Management techniques are those programs, procedures and strategies that assist you in performing one or more of the management functions. Specific techniques are presented in Parts II, III, and IV. A skill is proficiency in a way of doing something using your hands, body and brain. Thus the management skills are those personal abilities the manager uses in achieving results through the technical mode and the human mode. Such skills include communicating (via one's behavior, body language, eye contact, facial expression, listening, reading, silence, speaking, touching, writing), conceptualizing, decision making, discussion leading, instructing, improving methods, managing time, motivating, perceiving, and problem solving. In summary, managerial performance skills are the ways in which a nurse manager utilizes management techniques to effectively carry out the management functions of planning, doing and controlling.

Environmental Influences

A variety of environmental factors also influence you in your job. These factors range from the patients themselves to members of the medical staff, members of the nursing department, other employees throughout the hospital, visitors and so on. Environmental factors are such groups as business, community, educational, governmental, labor, political, professional, religious, social and volunteer organizations. These groups exert a variety of economic, cultural and behavioral pressures on your healthcare agency too. These groups and the people who represent them influence you directly and indirectly whether or not you have regular personal contact with them. They have an impact on your apperceptive mass. They influence your decision making, consciously or subconsciously. As a nurse manager you need to be aware of the environmental factors so that you can give them the attention they deserve, appropriate to decision making at your organizational level. Such factors become increasingly significant as you progress to higher levels of responsibility in any organizational setting.

The admonition to consider the environmental factors implies the necessity for a balanced interpretation of what they mean and how they should influence decisions and actions. This is complicated by the fact that we human beings are unable to be purely objective in interpreting what we see. John Ross, an Australian researcher, reports that the human perceptual system draws on unconscious interpretation of visual data and decides what to see. One research finding indicated that we apparently idealize what we see. Psychologist Ross believes that the visual system may have a program, an arrangement for perceiving shapes in time and space. "What we see is an interpretation. We adopt a perceptual attitude in order to comprehend the world."[3]

Most of us recognize from our own experience the selective receptivity of our senses. When we listen, somehow we often hear what we want to hear and screen out the rest. When we try to identify our feelings, we may be shocked to learn of our seeming inability (or unwillingness) to recognize and express our feelings—as contrasted to our thoughts. We may have difficulty even in recognizing the existence and influence of the affective and cognitive components in learning, teaching, decision making, interpersonal relations and patient care. When we do discover the productive balanced interrelationship of feeling and thinking, of heart and mind, (through transactional analysis, a learning laboratory, an ACT-U-AR, or similar experience) then our lives and work may become more satisfying.

This discussion has been an exercise in conceptualizing your workworld. Conceptual ability is a vital mental skill in your work as a nurse and a manager. A concept is an idea. It exists within your own apperceptive mass, the associational areas of your brain. A concept may be considered a general understanding, thought, or notion that grows out of specific instances or occurrences. We recognize that your workworld can never be as carefully structured, uniformly balanced, or as static a concept as described. On the contrary, it is more like a changing, dynamic, freewheeling, psychedelic, multi-dimensional kind of a world. Every manager has to conceptualize this big picture, to be familiar with its details and how they fit together, and perceive how the meaning of that picture affects day-to-day problem solving and decision making.

THE PERFORMANCE DESCRIPTION

The use of job descriptions has been the traditional way of describing the duties of the person holding a particular job. We much prefer "performance" descriptions and encourage their use at every opportunity. A performance description has some similarities to a job description, but the two are basically different because they are developed for two different purposes. The job description, by its very title, describes a job. It is prepared by a process of job analysis and its purpose is primarily to provide the necessary descriptive job information for job evaluation purposes. Supplemental uses include orienting a new person to a job and, to some extent, for assistance in recruitment.

A performance description, by contrast, describes performance responsibilities. It is prepared by a process of performance analysis carried out initially by employees with their own managers. Its purpose is to reach agreement and understanding, between superior and subordinate, regarding the subordinate's performance resposibilities so that meaningful ongoing self-evaluation of performance can take place. The emphasis in the preparation and use of a performance description is in reaching a mutual understanding between superior and subordinate regarding who is to do what for whom, when and how well—so that there can be later understanding and agreement regarding what was done for whom, when and how well. A further examination of these purposes is included in Part III dealing with results-oriented performance evaluation.

The head nurse example (Appendix G, page 305) is used because it is representative of a performance description for any nurse-manager. The descriptions for other nursing personnel, either at the staff nurse level or at higher levels of management responsibility, are similar in form and partially similar in content. First of all, the description provides a simple statement of the purpose of the person in the head nurse position. The major performance responsibilities are listed on the left side of the sheet. These responsibilities are grouped according to the persons for whom they are carried out. Performance responsibilities are always activities that are done for someone else. On the right side of the sheet are statements for each item of responsibility that indicate the measurable conditions which will exist when performance is satisfactory. Thus the head nurse has a responsibility to his or her own nurse manager to "help with budgetary planning and operate the unit within the budget." Performance is satisfactory when "the budget is realistically related to patient care programs and expenses are within the budget." A full examination of these performance descriptions will help to complete the picture of the workworld of the nurse manager. (See Appendix G for an example of a Head Nurse performance description and see Appendix A for a lengthier example of a performance description entitled "General Performance Responsibilities of Administrative and Management Personnel.")

GOALS AND RESPONSIBILITIES

The organizational chart of a department of nursing presents the structure of the department in terms of lines of authority and responsibilities among the members of the department. If you have not seen the organization chart for your department, you should obtain one and review it. Such a chart of organization is another important dimension in your understanding of your workworld.

Every organization exists for a purpose. This purpose is stated in the articles of incorporation, and is often elaborated in the form of a number of specific goals. The broad organizational goals must be translated into departmental and unit goals and objectives. The section on "Management by Objectives" in Part III presents the technique for carrying out such a program. all employees need to understand the goals and objectives of their department and their roles in carrying out the objectives. This concept is diagrammed in the MBO Schematic Organizational Plan (See Figure 3:2 in Chapter 3). The Financial Organization Chart (Figure 6:1 in Chapter 6) emphasizes another important aspect of organization. Everyone knows that everything that happens in an organization costs money. Too few members of the typical nursing department, however, know just how much money is being spent. Usually this is through no fault of the staff members themselves, but it does reflect upon agency administration.

As patients, we have had occasion to ask a variety of members of the patient care staff such questions as, "How much is my daily room charge? How much does it cost to provide me with the daily change of bed linen? Why does the bed linen have to be changed daily when I am ambulatory? Would my bill be less if my bed linen were not changed daily?" Response to such questions is usually a shrug of the shoulders, a guess, or an "I don't know." Such lack of knowledgeable response (and the absence of any apparent interest in the questions) is a sad commentary upon those hospitals' management and nursing leadership in today's healthcare world.

Nurse managers in a modern healthcare setting must be cost conscious themselves and help every staff person to be aware that everything he or she does has direct impact upon the expenses of running the department. Such an attitude is important to patient care. In our experience, appropriate emphasis on the financial aspects of nursing contributes to, rather than detracts from, patient care goals.

There is no need to overdramatize here the great significance of this subject of healthcare costs. Professional publications, the daily newspaper and other media regularly draw attention to the staggering increases in the cost of healthcare. The day-to-day operating expenses can be controlled best by those who provide the care. Nurse managers have a vital role in this. As a group, the nurse managers in healthcare agencies have responsibility for spending more of the agency budget than the managers in any other department. This responsibility has had too little emphasis in the past in terms of sound management practices. The chapter on annual budgetary planning provides specific help in this area.

THE NURSING PROCESS AND THE MANAGEMENT PROCESS

During recent decades a great amount of attention has been devoted to defining the practice of nursing. These efforts have been complicated by the variety of changes that have kept nursing in a state of flux. Within a single generation, nurses have seen their responsibilities analyzed, subdivided, broadened, delimited, reorganized, unionized and role-expanded so often that nurses can be forgiven if their view of nursing at times seemed cloudy and uncertain.

During this period, however, a clearly-defined and well-accepted framework for nursing emerged. This framework is the nursing process. The process includes four phases: assessing, planning, implementing, evaluating. While the nursing process is an excellent and useful conceptualization of what nurses do, too often the process is not understood or practiced successfully by the nurses themselves. Reasons for this vary, but include educational, organizational and philosophical deficiencies. Our purpose now is to compare the nursing process to the management process and identify the common source of each.

Ruth Mrozek makes a useful comparison by showing how the nursing process and the problem-oriented charting system are modelled on the pattern of the scientific method.[4] This is the problem-finding, problem-solving pattern of (1) gathering and interpreting information so that a problem can be clearly defined; (2) considering alternatives for action, making a decision, and developing an action plan; (3) implementing the plan; (4) evaluating the results, and continuing the cycle of progress toward meeting the patient's problems and needs.

The accompanying diagram of Figure 1:1 portrays the parallel patterns and cyclical relationship of the nursing process, the problem-oriented charting system and the scientific method. The three cyclical models are set in the integrative concept of the basic management functions of planning, doing and controlling. Clearly, the four steps of the scientific method are the core of this diagram. After the term "scientific management" became popular early in this century, it was often described as the four steps of planning, organizing, directing and controlling. We have used the simpler modern version of three basic functions of the management process shown in the figure as the encompassing cycle that is our theme.

This model is introduced at this point because it is so fundamental to the conceptual structure which we are building with you. Later chapters elaborate upon the various elements of the model. One of the reasons that many good nurses perform so well as good nurse managers is that they have been so well educated in the use of the scientific method. Scientific management is based soundly in the scientific method. And the essence of scientific management is measurement plus control. Clearly the nursing process and the problem-oriented nursing system are specific applications of the management, or scientific, process. The framework for nursing today and tomorrow has evolved beyond the nursing process per se. The nursing process is a component of the problem-oriented nursing system (PONS) which in turn is a necessary part of the patient care process (see Table 2:1 in Chapter 2). The components of PONS, in nurse-management terminology, involve the selective adaptation and use of functions, techniques and skills directed toward meeting patient/client needs.

THE TRANSITION TO MANAGER

The difference between being a *nurse* manager and a nurse *manager* is more than a matter of semantics. A primary nurse working with a limited number of patients uses the management process in providing and managing the care of those patients. The emphasis is on a personal application of the nursing process while providing guidance and leadership to other members of the patient care team as a secondary responsibility. A head nurse, however, or a patient care coordinator responsible for several units, necessarily has to place major emphasis on the personnel management aspects of the work. Clinical skills are still necessary and important, but the management skills must at the very least be of equal importance.

The career change from being a professional nurse to becoming a professional nurse manager is a big step. For many persons it is the most significant step in a nursing career. The nurse manager is still a member of a patient care team. But now, instead of being one of many persons under the direction of someone else, the manager is the someone else—the person in charge of and responsible for coordinating the work of the other team members (in a unit, section or department). It is a change from a job status which is primarily one of doing the work oneself to one which involves getting work done through others.

Involved here is a basic change in one's way of thinking. The

Figure 1:1
An Integrative Functional Comparison
of
Process, Method, and System

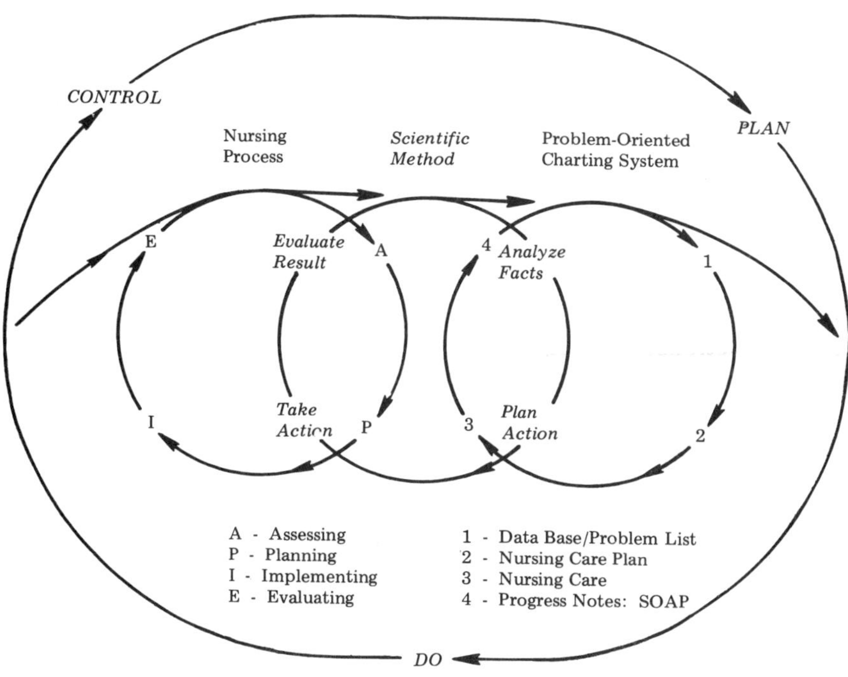

manager can no longer think only in terms of my work and my job. The manager's concern is about our work and our jobs. No longer are you responsible just for your own work, facilities and equipment. Now you are responsible for the work, facilities and equipment of all the nursing personnel on your unit. You may even feel that you have assumed responsibility for the people themselves, your most important asset outside of yourself. And in a way you have. But in another sense you have been given an opportunity to help your people become more responsible for themselves. This opportunity is one of your greatest challenges. It can be met through the ways you shape the working environment and personnel relationships, the ways in which you utilize your human-mode and technical-mode skills. It can mean using the job enrichment concept described by M. Scott Myers in *Every Employee A Manager.*[5] Myers explains how the customary ideas about what a manager does (planning, organizing, leading, controlling) compared with the traditional role of the worker (doing manual labor) has contributed to the management/labor gap.

In the traditional organization this view of role relationships has been held by managers and workers alike. Managers are the ones who have been presumed to have the maturity, knowledge, ability and responsibility to plan, direct and control what the workers do. And the members of the labor force appear to have been perceived as uninformed, immature, irresponsible and less intelligent. The result of these commonly held views about the role of managers as compared with the role of the labor group has led to understandable feelings of social distance, of alienation, of differing needs and concerns. While a certain amount of such feelings may seem inevitable, many modern managers are finding ways to decrease such feelings and to close the management/labor gap.

Myers comments upon the role of labor unions in formalizing and widening the gap between the employer and the employees. But he sees two major forces at work to close or eliminate the gap between labor and management. One such force is the rising socio-economic status of the less privileged members of the employee group, accompanied by rising expectations. The second force is an increasing awareness and acceptance by managers of the democratic pattern in organizational leadership. Myers presents his concept of the enriched job for all employees—not just the manager group—as one that includes the planning and control functions as well as the doing (Fig. 1:2).

This is a way to encourage and permit more employees to think for themselves. It encourages more creativity. It permits a wider range of doing. It places more trust in the employee. It builds more interest,

Figure 1:2
Meaningful Work Model

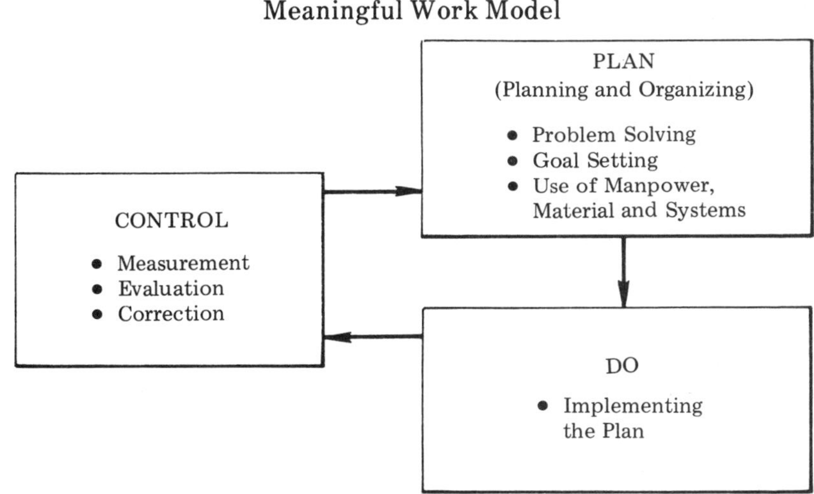

From M. Scott Myers, *Every Employee A Manager* (New York: McGraw-Hill, 1970), p.70. Used with permission from McGraw-Hill Book Co.

self respect and pride. In short, job enrichment as envisioned here helps each person to meet more fully his own needs through, and because of, achieving more successfully the agency and patient objectives.

As a professional nurse you may never have experienced the feeling of being on the labor side of the management/labor gap. But if you have had that experience at any time during your career, so much the better. It can assist you in having greater empathy for your employees at all job levels. And it may encourage you to learn more of the leadership skills and management techniques that permit all employees to use their maximum capabilities in the kind of enriched job structure that leads to greater self direction, self control and accountability as well as better patient care.

A hospital provides a natural setting for the application of the job enrichment concept. In nursing, many persons already have the experience of managing their own jobs. It is implicit in the earlier discussion of the parallel models of the nursing process and the management process. But nonnurses usually have not been trained in the four steps of the nursing process, and do not have the privilege of using it. And many nurses do not use it either. This may be due to their own lack of initiative or because of the kind of leadership they receive. Some nursing administrators do an injustice to themselves, their patients and their staff members by placing too little emphasis on the nursing process, the problem-oriented system and team-building using modern management concepts. Often such administrators understand and agree with the need for these things but fail to implement them successfully because of a blockage in the affective area (emotions and feelings), or because of a leadership style that is too firmly fixed at the authoritarian end of the scale. Such a style is characterized by telling, in contrast to the facilitating behavior of a goal-oriented leader. Between these two styles are varying degrees of selling and involving.

Authoritarian leaders tend to make their own decisions with a minimum of consultation. They tell staff members what to do and how to do it or they try to sell their people on a course of action. They seek prompt compliance and obedience. Goal-oriented leaders usually involve their people in problem solving and decision making whenever possible. They seek self direction and responsibility from staff members. They are facilitative managers in the sense of making themselves available for help, materials, information—for whatever the staff members need for patient care purposes, for doing satisfactory and satisfying work. The most skillful managers (whether authority-oriented or goal-oriented by inclination) are able to use the basic appropriate combination of telling, selling, involving and facilitating as suitable to the needs of particular situations.

A nurse manager's leadership style is affected strongly by the kind of bosses he or she has had in the past and who provided early role models. Another influence is the kind of transition the nurse manager achieved in moving from staff nursing into management. For most persons, the necessary change in one's way of thinking referred to earlier does not happen automatically. It has to be learned. Habit patterns are strong. New habits and skills—managerial habits and skills—must be developed and used. Admittedly, professional nurses are likely to make the transition to manager more easily than other healthcare workers. Nurses have carried legal responsibility for their actions and the actions of those co-workers whom they direct. Nurses have learned to understand and accept personal responsibility and liability. Yet when nurses elect to shift from the clinical track to the management track, an adjustment in orientation and performance becomes necessary. Part of the adjustment involves regular reading of management literature. This includes such periodicals as *The Journal of Nursing Administration, Supervisor Nurse, Modern Healthcare* and *Health Care Management Review.*

As a nurse manager you may also wish to expand your membership in professional associations to include such groups as the Society for

Advancement of Management, the American Society for Training and Development, or the Association for Humanistic Psychology. Like many other nurse managers you will discover that selective reading of management journals and books and active participation in one or more management groups helps with your own self development as a manager, consciously directs your attention to broad management problems and ways of resolving them, and assists in your change in thinking from professional clinical nurse to professional nurse manager — your big step.

As a manager, you have to get the right things done at the right time through and with the right people. Your focus is on productive action as a manager achieving desired results through people. These words are just as meaningful for a director of nursing service and a hospital administrator as they are for a new unit nurse manager. Fully understood, this generalized definition of your purpose means that you have to meet patient care goals by guiding the nursing staff into effective action, helping your people to attain agency objectives, aiding your people to satisfy their own personal needs, counselling with staff members regarding their performance results, encouraging people to greater self-development and growth, and allowing the staff to use their creative talents.

Surveys and interviews conducted with agency personnel at all levels have told us what their concerns are. These concerns include just about everything from benefits, communications, and job satisfaction to supervisory relations, training, and unions. But there are five which are mentioned most frequently, especially by technical and professional people.

These major concerns are:

1. Relations Between Nurse Manager and Nursing Staff: General rapport; performance reviews; professional guidance.

2. Wage and Salary Administration: Hiring pay vs. pay for performance; understanding agency policy; merit vs. general increases.

3. Mobility: Opportunities for advancement, reassignment and transfer.

4. Utilization: Good use of education, experience, and abilities; a chance to make a contribution.

5. Recognition: Sense of status; a feeling that my boss knows my worth as a person, and shows it.

These are vital concerns — for the staff, the organization and patients. Better understanding and improvements can occur only with the help of every individual nurse manager and others with agency leadership responsibility.

THE NEW WORLD OF MANAGER-EMPLOYEE RELATIONS

Lets's face it; it's a changing world we live in. For some of us, it changes too fast; for others not fast enough. Some see the changes as for the better; others see them as for the worse. Some of us adapt readily to change; others find it more difficult. But saddest of all are those who appear to see no change; or who, seeing it, recognize no need to adapt to it. One of the significant changes that affects your job as a nurse manager has to do with the nature of those persons you must lead today. Consider today's new generation of employees. Compared with an older generation, your newer staff members tend to be better educated with higher levels of technical knowledge; they have a higher sense of security and high expectations; they question older- generation values; they see interpersonal relations as either open, honest and trusting — or as characterized by suspicion, dishonesty and distrust; they may view managers as restrictive and exploitative; they resist manipulation, seek involvement and take pride in individual accomplishment; they desire to use their full range of abilities and are hostile toward a confining job environment; and they are unwilling to adapt to hypocritical standards of behavior and value concepts.

These facts of your employee environment, together with other changes you can identify, mean that your job as a nurse manager is likely to be challenging and exciting. Sometimes your people will be aggravating to work with and difficult to manage, but they will be interesting and exciting to lead. They will respond, create, grow and help you — given the opportunity. Most will take responsibility, and you can hold them accountable for it. They'll do a good job for you — if you give them a good job to do. If you are newly promoted as a nurse manager, you are likely to be more fully responsive to the opinions, needs and feelings of your people now than you will be ever again. One reason for this is that you have so recently been one of them. The coming weeks, months, and years will involve you more and more in concerns of nursing management — objectives, costs, budgets, reports, conferences, quality — to mention a few. These may tend to lessen your responsiveness to your people and their needs for feeling secure, respected, recognized, worthwhile, growing. Protect yourself against this usual trend, since your real success as a nurse manager will come from being able to help your people satisfy their goals and needs through the process of contributing to unit and departmental objectives. You have to do it your own way. That's first. Be true to yourself. Don't try to fit into someone else's mold. At the same time, don't miss opportunities to learn better ways to manage. Sharpen your leadership skills. Learn from others. Learn by practicing the best method. For example, here's something to add to your management tool kit right know. Use it the next time you have a problem to resolve. Make it part of the usual steps of getting facts, defining the problem, developing alternative solutions, taking action, and follow through.

Problems are caused by persons who...
• Don't Know — and who need — Job Knowledge
• Can't Do — and who need — Job Skills
• Don't Care — and who need — Self-motivation, through need satisfaction.

Problems are resolved by persons who...
• Consult with others for facts, feelings, opinions;
• Explore the problem (ask, listen, discuss);
• Agree upon what will be done;
• Set objectives (for achievement)
• Set a date (for completion)
• Evaluate (for results).

You learn by doing, especially when you practice the best method. These simple steps, and their more complete presentation in subsequent pages, can help you to:

• Relate and respond to the persons you lead, to recognize and build upon their value systems, dislike of hypocrisy, desire for a sense of community, contribution and achievement.
• Contribute to improved handling of major concerns of your people: supervisory-subordinate relations (rapport through rapping, honest goal-oriented performance reviews, self-development guidance); salary administration (pay increases when deserved; explanation of reasons when not possible); utilization (achieving full people-potential by making good use of their education and special abilities); recognition (overt action, regularly, to help others meet their needs for status and sense of self worth).
• Perform your management functions — planning, doing, controlling — most effectively.

THE TRADEMARKS OF A REAL PROFESSIONAL

What makes a person a real professional? Are you a real pro in your field? We decided a few years ago to establish for ourselves a set of criteria having general applicability in any field of human endeavor.

Then, at rare intervals, we have awarded a suitably engraved certificate to qualifying persons. An accompanying letter includes an appropriate explanation. While originally inspired by a touch of whimsy, we are entirely serious about the significance of the criteria and the award. We hope that you, the reader, feel that you are ready to qualify as a real professional nurse manager — or that the time will come when you will advise us that you are so qualified to receive the award and the following message:

> You are cordially welcomed as a newly elected member of PRO, the Realistic Order of Professionals. Your name has been inscribed in the Great Book of the Order, recording for posterity this well-deserved honor and recognition. Henceforth and forevermore you, as A REAL PRO, are entitled to use after your name the distinctive designation reserved for members of the Order in good standing: PRO. May you always continue to exemplify in your life and work the characteristics that have led to your nomination and acceptance into the fellowship of the Order.

Trademarks of a Real Professional

Knowledge: You know your field of activity thoroughly. You have studied and worked to gain your knowledge and are not likely to be fooled or bluffed about your field.

Experience: You have much meaningful experience. You have been exposed to the tough situations and can react spontaneously with the right response.

Skill: You are an expert. You do a top quality job. You out-perform the amateurs. You have learned the best method, practiced it, and can deliver in the pinches.

Confidence: Your abilities and knowledge have bred a justifiable confidence. It shows. Others respect it. Your confidence is not only in yourself, but in your fellow team workers.

Mobility: You are fully mobile. You are secure in your ability, and have no concern for job security as such. You are welcome on anybody's team.

Performance: You like to win. You use all of your talents to come out on top, to get the results you can be proud of.

Recognition: You get much satisfaction from your work, and you are realistic about your own worth. You know that adequate compensation takes many forms.

Leadership: You are willing to provide leadership in your field, devoting a portion of your time and effort to this end, to be known as a giver rather than a taker. You see the value and need of service *pro bono publico.*

NOTES

1. Lawrence Appley, *A Management Concept* (New York: American Management Association, 1969), p. 59.
2. Joan and Warren Ganong with John Huenefeld, "Motive Force: A Key to Evaluating Nurse Managers," *J. Nursing Administration,* 4 (July-August, 1974), p. 17-19.
3. John Ross, "The Resources of Binocular Perception," *Scientific American,* 234, 3 (March, 1976), p. 80-86.
4. Ruth Mrozek, "Incorporating the Nursing Process into the Problem-Oriented Record" in H.K. Walker, MD; J.W. Hurst, MD; and M.F. Woody, RN; eds. *Applying the Problem-Oriented System* (New York:Medcom Press, 1973), 355-357.
5. M. Scott Myers, *Every Employee A Manager* (New York:McGraw-Hill, Inc., 1970), pp. 55-95.

SUGGESTED READINGS

Books

Argyris, Chris. *Personality and Organization* (New York: Harper & Row, 1957).

Arndt, Clara and Huckabay, Loucine. *Nursing Administration: Theory for Practice with a Systems Approach*   (St. Louis: C.V. Mosby Co., 1975).

Beyers, M., and Phillips, C. *Nursing Management for Patient Care* (Boston: Little, Brown & Co., 1971).

Combs, A.W., Avila, D.L.; and Purkey, W.W. *Helping Relationships: Basic Concepts for the Helping Professions* (Boston: Allyn and Bacon, 1971).

Cunningham, R.N., Jr. *Governing Hospitals: Trustees and the New Accountabilities* (Chicago: American Hospital Association, 1975).

DiVincenti, Marie. *Administering Nursing Service* (Boston: Little, Brown & Co., 1972).

Drucker, Peter. *Management: Tasks, Responsibilities, Practices* (New York: Harper & Row, 1974).

Drucker, Peter. *The Effective Executive* (New York: Harper & Row, 1966).

Frankel, Victor. *Man's Search for Meaning* (New York: Simon & Shuster, 1970).

Ganong, Joan and Warren. *HELP for the Head Nurse: A Management Guide*, 2nd ed., (Chapel Hill, N.C.: W.L. Ganong Co., 1975).

Geitgey, Doris A. *A Handbook for Head Nurses* (Philadelphia: F.A. Davis Co., 1971).

Goble, Frank. *Excellence in Leadership* (New York: American Management Association, 1972).

Goble, Frank. *The Third Force: The Psychology of Abraham Maslow* (New York: Grossman Publishers, 1970).

Haimann, Theo. *Supervisory Management for Health Care Institutions* (St. Louis: The Catholic Hospital Assoc., 1973).

Hampden-Turner, Charles. *Radical Man* (Cambridge, Mass.; Schankman Publishing, 1970).

Hersey, Paul, and Blanchard, Ken. *Management of Organizational Behavior*, 2nd ed. (Englewood Cliffs, N.J.: Prentice-Hall, 1972).

Herzberg, Frederick; Mausner, Bernard; Peterson, Richard O.; and Capwell, Dora F. *Job Attitudes: Review of Research Opinion* (Pittsburgh: Psychological Service of Pittsburgh, 1957).

Jourard, Sidney. *The Transparent Self* (Princeton, N. J.: Van Nostrand Co., Insight Book, 1964).

Jourard, Sidney. *Personal Adjustment* (New York: MacMillan Co., 1963).

Kraegel, Janet et al. *Patient Care Systems* (Philadelphia: J. B. Lippincott Co., 1974).

Kriegel, Julia. *The Head Nurse: Thoughts and Decisions* (New York: MacMillan and Co., 1968).

Likert, Rensis. *The Human Organization: Its Management and Value* (New York: McGraw-Hill, Inc., 1967).

Marriner, Ann. *The Nursing Process* (St. Louis: The C.V. Mosby Company, 1975).

Maslow, Abraham. *Eupsychian Management* (Homewood, Ill.: The Dorsey Press, 1965).

Maslow, Abraham. *The Farther Reaches of Human Nature* (New York: The Viking Press, 1971).

Maslow, Abraham. *Motivation and Personality* 2nd ed. (New York: Harper & Row, 1970).

Maslow, Abraham. *Toward a Psychology of Being* (Princeton: Van Nostrand, Insight Books, 1968).

Maher, John, ed. *New Perspectives in Job Enrichment*(New York: Van Nostrand Reinhold Co., Frontiers in Management Series, 1971).

McGregor, Douglas. *The Human Side of Enterprise* (New York: McGraw-Hill, Inc., 1960).

Myers, M. Scott. *Every Employee A Manager: More Meaningful Work Through Job Enrichment* (New York:McGraw-Hill, Inc., 1970).

Orem, Dorothea. *Nursing: Concepts of Practice* (New York: McGraw-Hill, Inc., 1971).

Ornstein, Robert. *The Psychology of Consciousness* (San Francisco: W.H. Freeman, 1972).

Powell, John. *Why Am I Afraid To Tell You Who I Am?* (Niles, Ill.: Argus Communications, 1969).

Simon, Sidney et al. *Values Clarification* (New York: Hart Publishing Co., 1972).

Stevens, Barbara J. *The Nurse as Executive* (Wakefield, Mass.: Contemporary Publishing, 1975).

Walker, H. Kenneth, MD; Hurst, J. Willis, MD, and Woody, Mary F., RN, eds., *Applying the Problem-Oriented System* (New York: Medcom Press, 1973).

Articles

Aydelotte, Myrtle, "Administration and Directors of Nursing," *Hospitals*, 48 (December 16, 1974), pp. 61-63.

Bennett, Addison, "New Thinking Required for Development of Management Effectiveness," *Hospitals*, 50 (February 16, 1976), pp. 67-70.

Ferguson, Marilyn, ed., *Brain-Mind Bulletin* (Los Angeles: Interface Press), Published semimonthly. This bulletin may be obtained from the publisher, P. O. Box 42211, Los Angeles, Calif. 90042.

Ganong, Joan and Warren, "Are Head Nurses Obsolete?"*Journal of Nursing Administration* 5 (September 1975), pp. 16-18.

Ganong, Warren L. and Joan Mary, "Good Advice: Coping with the Changing Role of the Nurse," *Journal of Nursing Administration*, 2 (March-April, 1972), p. 8.

Kinsella, Cynthia, "Nursing," *Hospitals*, 49 (April 1, 1975), pp. 101-105.

Nuckolls, Katherine B., "Who Decides What the Nurse Can Do?" *Nursing Outlook*, 22 (October 1974), pp. 626-631.

Part II

Patient Care Management

Chapter 2
The Problem-Oriented Nursing System

THE CONCEPTUAL FRAMEWORK

The tides of change in our healthcare system affect everyone. Nurses especially feel the impact of new demands upon healthcare agencies. Nurses have to do something about meeting the more stringent accreditation requirements, standards imposed as a result of federally funded services, nursing audit, cost containment, budgetary planning, PSRO, POMR, HMO, unionization, inflation, national health insurance, community accountability, and all the rest. And nurses have to maintain their professional integrity and personal commitment to patient care while coping with the welter of wonderful work.

This is, in fact, a time of unprecedented opportunity for nurses. It is a time when, as perhaps never before, nurses are being invited to take new initiatives in many areas of service and organizational leadership. It is a time when all nurses in whatever role — as clinician, manager or educator — can more fully utilize their full range of talents, knowledge and skills. It is also a time to maintain perspective, to take a balanced view of what nurses — yourself, in particular — should do, can do, and want to do.

It may be timely to set aside some quiet time with yourself to take stock of your life situation. Consider where you have come from, where you are, and where you want to go. Ask yourself, "What do I want to do with my career as a nurse?" We believe that most of us can do what we want to do if we want it badly enough — enough to do what is necessary to achieve a goal that is worthwhile to us. The introspection that is necessary for you to explore your life/work goals is likely to lead to identifying and examining your values and motivation, your knowledge and skills — those components of your apperceptive mass as reviewed in Part I. This is quite appropriate as a kind of backdrop for PONS, the subject of this chapter. Choices are available to nurses as never before. The options are many. And the means exist for implementing personal and group objectives. Becoming an effective nurse manager is, for many nurses, both a conscious career choice and a means toward an end. PONS can be one of the building blocks in the process of goal achievement for all nurses, whether on the clinical, management, or educational track.

While a wide range of opportunities are available to nurses, they exist within the structure of the healthcare delivery system in general and of the patient care process in particular. We view the patient care process as being composed of identifiable system elements with which every nurse should be familiar. These system elements provide the basis for both a medical model and a nursing model of patient care. To assist in a consistent use and understanding of terminology, here are definitions of some of the foregoing terms:

Process: A series of actions, changes, or functions that bring about a particular result.

Model: A tentative ideational structure used as a testing device; a means of communicating a concept.

System: A group of interrelated elements forming a collective entity.

Element: A fundamental, essential or irreducible constituent of a composite entity.

An accompanying diagram, Table 2:1, presents the patient care process and identifies the system elements, the medical model and the nursing model of patient care. This diagram presents a conceptual framework within which to view the patient care process from the time the person (client) enters the healthcare system as a hospital patient.

The system elements as shown in the center column of the illustration begin with the patient preadmission procedures and follow the patient through the steps of initial assessment of the patient and his related problems, the development of a plan of care and its implementation, followed by the evaluation of the patient's progress and problems. At the next level of the patient's progress is the identification of new problems and the revision of care plans together with their implementation and evaluation. This sequence, as indicated, is repeated as often as necessary during the patient's hospitalization. The next stages are indicated as the discharge procedure and referral to suitable followup care at home or through other agencies. The entire sequence—from initial admission to discharge and referral for home care—may be repeated as required by the patient's condition.

Table 2:1
The Patient Care Process: Comparison of Medical and Nursing Models of Patient Care

Medical Model	System Elements	Nursing Model
1. Assess patient, write initial orders	1. Patient preadmission procedures	1. Preadmission procedures
2. Write additional orders	2. Admission	2. Admit
3. History and physical exam	3. Assessment of patient	3. Initial patient interview & observation
4. Problem list	4. Problem identification	4. Problem list
5. Medical plan	5. Plan of care	5. Initial nursing plan & nursing directives
6. Order Rx, medications, record	6. Implementation of care plan	6. Give care, Rx, meds, teach, listen, observe, record, initiate discharge planning
7. Rounds, observe, confer	7. Evaluate problems & progress	7. Give care, rounds, observe, confer, coordinate
8. Write new orders, document on progress notes, Rx, medications, rounds, observe, confer	8. Identify new problems, adjust plan, implement adjusted plan, evaluate problems and progress	8. Revise care plan, write new nursing directives, Modify care appropriately & document on patient record, give care, rounds, observe, confer, coordinate
	REPEAT SEQUENCE 1 THROUGH 7	
9. Order	9. Discharge	9. Finalize discharge plans, write discharge summary, discharge
10. Write order, fill in referral forms	10. Referral	10. Write nursing directives, fill in referral forms
	11. Initial visit and assessment	11. Initial interview, observation, examination

REPEAT SEQUENCE 1 THROUGH 7 AS REQUIRED

The medical model shown in the left column of the illustration and the nursing model in the right column parallel the system elements as described. The medical model has its focus in the medical care of the patient, while the nursing model has its focus on nursing and other aspects of patient care for which the nursing department is responsible.

The model as presented is intended to be as simple as possible and yet provide a reasonably comprehensive conceptualization of the patient care process as it exists. As you review it in detail, ask yourself a number of questions about it. Are the system elements as presented consistent with the patient care process in your agency? Is the nursing model compatible with the system elements, based upon your own experience? Are the medical and nursing models correctly interrelated? As you ask these questions and any others that may occur to you, make a note of any exceptions, additions, or corrections that you believe are necessary to make the diagram an acceptable portrayal of the patient care process as you perceive it in your own agency. What other questions are stimulated by your consideration and discussion of the diagram? What additional ideas do you have regarding a more visionary model of what the patient care delivery system should be, as compared with how it is now?

The foregoing provides at least a beginning for, or some elaboration upon, your own conceptual framework for considering patient care, nursing and yourself in the dynamic healthcare environment of today and the immediate future. As you have considered this conceptual model and attempted to relate it to the workworld of the nurse manager as presented in Part I, you undoubtedly have seen some similarities to the management process and the responsibilities of nurse managers. If such is not the case, we recommend strongly that you review all of this material again to consider its implications not only for yourself as a nurse but also to yourself as a manager. This is important because the whole thrust of this book is to help you develop an integrated view of the patient care process and the management process so that they are seen as inseparable. Admittedly you may not yet have developed the habit of perceiving yourself in the managerial role. We believe that the sooner you do perceive yourself as a manager, the sooner will you — and nursing as a whole — be able to relate most successfully to the other members of the patient care team in meeting the identified needs and goals of patients.

Your reactions to the foregoing are very important. You may be feeling now that "this is not for me;" or you may be feeling that "this is really what I want." Your reactions are dictated largely by your own perception of yourself and your perception of nursing. You may think of yourself as just a nurse who carries out assigned tasks, procedures and routines for patients. You may see yourself as a patient care manager who works as a primary nurse with your individual patients to assist them in meeting their objectives through carrying out the medical care plan and the nursing care plan. Or you may see yourself as a nurse manager accepting full responsibility for clinical management, operations management and human resources management. If one of your reactions is, "Oh, I could never do that!" then you may feel restricted by what you believe to be personal liabilities and roadblocks to your own growth. Whether these are imagined or real, it is possible to know thyself while emphasizing the positive. It is a simple fact of self-development and of assisting with the development of others that you cannot build on personal liabilities. You can build only upon personal assets.

Certainly you must face problems that develop out of your own personal life/work situations and recognize their influence on your own goal achievement. But rather than focus on them as problems, you can elect, if you adopt a suitable frame of mind, to see problems as opportunities. When you do this — when you perceive a problem as an opportunity—you adopt a frame of mind (a "willing mind," to use a southern phrase) that helps to marshal your available resources, utilize your assets and skills, and make progress in spite of the problems. Roadblocks are viewed as temporary obstacles to be removed, not as barriers preventing your further progress.

We recognize that the performance of nurses and nurse/managers is influenced by their perceptions of their roles and of nursing, growing out of their education and experience. We recognize and bemoan the fact that in all-too-many situations, there tends to be a different emphasis in nursing education as compared with the emphasis found in nursing service. This is neither healthy nor desirable. To the student at any level there is much merit in a learning focus which emphasizes, "This is how it should be." And for the beginning nurse practitioner the emphasis for each working day is necessarily, "This is how it must be." We observe that nursing education faculties and nurse managers are increasing their efforts toward striking an appropriate balance between the two extremes. Even so, both groups need to place more emphasis on nursing as such, rather than upon education and service as the elements of a dichotomy. The dilemma of new staff nurses fresh from nursing education programs was summarized succinctly by Edith P. Lewis, editor of *Nursing Outlook*, who wrote: "To the student we say, 'This is your patient.' To the staff nurse, 'This is your job.' Small wonder that in the transition from the one to the other the nurse ends up by devaluing the patient, herself, and the job."[1] The role of education must continue to be not only the teaching of a philosophy, principles and skills of nursing, but also to provide the learning opportunities for the student to develop the personal skill of conceptualizing ideas and constructs. Part IV deals more fully with these matters. In the meantime, we can examine the contrasts in the two conceptualizations of the nursing role which Edith Lewis described so starkly.

One could be called the "Nursing Workload Concept" in which the patients are seen as generating a daily volume of routine work to be done through the performance of necessary tasks and procedures. This view is symbolized by the question sometimes heard on the nursing units, "Do you have your patients done yet?" In all of our experience as patients, we have never yet experienced a feeling of being "properly done" or "finished." We know of no patients who ever feel this way. Even allowing poetic license for the casualness of day-to-day working terminology, the question is an unfortunate one because it reflects the point of view, concept and philosophy of the patient-as-workload. Implicit in such a viewpoint is the idea that the purpose of nurses is to do things for patients — to carry out procedures, to perform tasks and to do all the routine work which is related to patient care. It is easy to understand how this viewpoint became common, not only among supervisors of past years, but also among modern nurse managers who have been under strong pressures to contain costs, reduce staffing and keep expenses within the budget. The trend toward measuring workload and work output over the past two decades has encouraged this workload concept.

The other concept, the "Patient Care Management Concept," presents an alternative way of viewing the nursing function. In this view the patient is seen as a person with identifiable needs and problems for which he seeks help. The patient (insofar as he is able to do so) participates with his doctor, his nurse and his family (or significant others) in developing the goals for his care, together with the objectives that must be met to achieve the goals. Where this concept prevails, the relevant day-to-day question is "How well is the patient meeting his objectives?"

The differences between these concepts are pronounced, not only as two views of nursing but also as they influence the day-to-day operations of patient care units. Procedures and task-oriented activities will continue to be necessary in the myriad aspects of providing patient care. But such activities should not become routines to be carried out for every patient regardless of need. For example:

> In a typical general hospital setting it is four o'clock in the morning. The night nurse discovers that Mr. Jones, a patient, has inadvertently pulled his drainage catheter apart and urine is running out into the bed. He is wet as are his pajamas and bedding. The nurse reconnects the catheter, washes up Mr. Jones and changes his pajamas and bedding. At seven o'clock there is a shift change and the night nurse goes off duty and another nurse comes on and is assigned to Mr. Jones. Immediately after breakfast Mr. Jones, in spite of his protests, is helped with a routine bath and a routine change of pajamas and bedding. In all likelihood around ten o'clock the head nurse asks the nurse assigned to Mr. Jones if he is "done yet." The things being "done" are carried out more as a daily routine than because of Mr. Jones' needs. The emphasis is on getting the morning routine "done" so that other routines can follow.

A routine may need to be established for a given patient — based upon his needs. But routines are not for everyone regardless of individual needs and desires. Such routines and the time, materials, tasks and people involved in them are wasteful and costly. In addition they may have little to do with the health status of patients like Mr. Jones.

One point that must be made here, however, is that over the years healthcare consumers have been programmed into expecting the routines when they become patients in general hospitals. More emphasis has been placed on the routines than upon the involvement of the patient in the planning of care designed to meet his needs and resolve his health problems. Nursing, with the support of administration, can help the consumer toward a better understanding of how nurses can contribute best to promoting health. Careful explanations and use of all aspects of the nursing process certainly help. Fortunately, there are hundreds of hospitals (an estimated 5% of all U.S. hospitals) now permitting and encouraging patients (who are able) to carry out for themselves all of of those activities—from activities of daily living to making their own beds—formerly done for them by nursing staff members or others. This trend needs to become the generally accepted norm in the best interests of the patient's health as well as for the economic health of the community at large.

Here are three summary statements growing out of the materials presented so far in this chapter which can serve as precepts for nurse managers:

1. Your perception of yourself as a person has great effect upon your behavior and aspirations in nursing.
2. Your view of nursing, (whether one of the two concepts mentioned or something in between, affects your role concept and the way you perform as a nurse.
3. Your understanding of the patient care process and of nursing as part of a system of patient care has profound influence upon your professional performance as a nurse manger.

PONS: AN OVERVIEW

The Problem-Oriented Nursing System and its components provide an integrated technique for the implementation of the "Patient Care Management Concept." PONS is a process for assessing, planning, implementing and evaluating patient care, based upon identified principles of nursing practice; involving the systematic recording of each patient's data base and identified problems; with an initial plan of care, progress notes, and discharge planning keyed to the problem list; supported by a nursing audit program, and with inservice and continuing education (for patients and staff) as a relevant component.

Such an approach to patient care that involves identifying the patient's needs and problems is not new. It has a long and highly respected history. A problem-oriented system has a specific connotation and is a fairly recent development. Dr. Lawrence L. Weed, the pioneer who began the development of the Problem-Oriented Medical System (POMS) and the Problem-Oriented Medical Record (POMR) in the 1950s at the University of Vermont College of Medicine, gained renown for his research and developmental work, and for his tireless teaching, speaking and counselling with all who would listen. His efforts led to gradual acceptance of POMS among his colleagues in medicine and to widespread acclaim by other professional groups — including nurses.[2]

The problem-oriented system as envisioned and developed by Dr. Weed provides for the use of the problem-oriented record by all members of the healthcare team. The introduction of this system, however, has lagged or not been attempted at all in many healthcare agencies where the medical staff has had no interest in initiating it. In the meantime, the many workshops, books and successful applications of the problem-oriented system have been educating more and more healthcare professionals to the benefits it offers for patient care. It is understandable that considerable frustration has existed among some professional groups in situations where they have long awaited leadership from the medical staff in introducing the problem-oriented system. Nurses in particular have wanted to participate in the initiation of the problem-oriented system. Now PONS provides a way for nurses to initiate the system within their own area of responsibility. PONS was developed out of nursing's need for a complete problem-oriented system. The efforts of many nursing departments contributed to PONS as a response to the need.

PONS incorporates a problem-oriented nursing record and the nursing process within a comprehensible system. The system, when introduced unilaterally by the nursing department, can stand on its own, assist in meeting documentation requirements and the standards for the patient's record, contribute to improved patient care and provide increased support for the members of the medical staff. PONS is so designed that it can be integrated easily with POMS and POMR when the medical staff adopts them. Or, lacking such adoption, PONS simply may continue indefinitely as the basic model for nursing — using a problem-oriented nursing record and the other components that contribute to optimum patient care.

The benefits are many. Many nurses who have assisted in implementing PONS have found that, for the first time, they have been able to develop a meaningful conceptual framework within which to view all of their efforts, whether as clinical nurses, nurse managers, or nurse educators. One of the reasons for this is the fact that PONS includes a number of components which once received lip service rather than committed application but which now have become, or may soon become, mandatory. These include nursing audit, complete nursing care plans as part of patients' records, greater recognition of patients' rights and legally valid documentation. Another important feature of PONS is its contribution toward the implementation of an effective results-oriented employee performance evaluation program (ROPEP). This is covered in considerable detail in Part III. One of the most gratifying aspects of PONS is the fact that so many nurses who have participated in its implementation in their own agencies have said, "For the very first time, I now feel that I am doing professional nursing!"

PONS: BASIC COMPONENTS OF THE SYSTEM

An accompanying illustration presents the five basic components of PONS together with the elements that make up each. The five components are:

1. The Foundation
2. The Process
3. The Problem-Oriented Nursing Record
4. Nursing Audit
5. Education

I. FOUNDATION

PRINCIPLES OF NURSING PRACTICE
Goals
Objectives
Definitions
Functions
Education
Research
Philosophy

Measure against the standards
Identify
Deficiencies & Strengths

V. EDUCATION
PATIENT & PERSONNEL
Patient
Teaching & Learning
Correct
Discrepancies
BUILD on
Strengths
Personnel
Inservice &
Continuing Education

You may find much that is familiar to you in the explanation of these components. This is as it should be. PONS is not something new and drastically different from what some well-run nursing departments have been doing for many years. Nursing audit, as a management technique (for that's what it really is), is relatively new in its actual application. The problem-oriented nursing record is perhaps the newest component for most nursing departments. But as we have indicated, the basis for this type of nursing record has been available for quite some time. The other components—which include the principles of nursing practice, the nursing process and education for both patients and staff—are much more familiar. A major contribution of PONS is the fact that it brings together all of the components in a meaningful way so that the whole becomes much more than the sum of all its parts. The meaning of the traditional components is enhanced by the addition of the new components. And the newer components, the problem-oriented record and the nursing audit, take on much greater significance when used in the context of the other three. Thus PONS provides the synergy to achieve optimum patient care. In fact, it sometimes provides a professional model which helps to motivate some members of a medical staff to take an active interest in the problem-oriented medical record. This is, of course, the ultimate test of success—when something works so well that others see its advantages and decide to adopt it for themselves.

The Foundation For PONS

The problem-oriented nursing system is structured upon a firm foundation of six elements: goals, objectives, definitions, functions, education and research. Underlying these elements, sometimes referred to as principles of nursing practice, is the basic philosophy (beliefs, values, precepts) that serves as a guide to action and conduct. The foundation for PONS may be seen as a set of firmly interlocked building blocks of these six elements on a base of philosophy.

A statement of one's philosophy is necessarily a personal, individualized expression of the beliefs and values by which one lives. It reflects a person's heritage and early training, education, life experiences and contemplation of the meaning of what one has learned.

The statement of philosophy for a healthcare agency expresses the beliefs and values by which the organization lives. By definition, a corporation is a body of persons granted a charter legally recognizing them as a separate entity having its own rights, privileges and liabilities. Thus the philosophy of a hospital, HMO, nursing home or similar agency is written by a person (or group of people) and reflects that person's (or group's) personal philosophy and views as to the beliefs, values and precepts that will serve as the guides to action and behavior for all who work for or serve the agency.

Sometimes the organizational philosophy is available in writing as a separate statement. Sometimes it is included in the organizational charter, the legal document issued by a govermental authority creating the corporation and defining its rights and privileges. When not otherwise available in writing, the people in an organization must interpret its philosophy from the pronouncements, actions and behavior of the recognized leader, the top person.

How important is your philosophy, and the philosophy of the leaders in your place of employment? Answers will vary. In Will Durant's introduction to his durable classic, *The Mansions of Philosophy*, he describes graphically the impact of change upon us all and the value of a philosophical outlook:

> All things flow, and we are at a loss to find some mooring and stability in the flux...we fear the experts in every field, and keep ourselves, for safety's sake, lashed to our narrow specialties. Everyone knows his part, but is ignorant of its meaning in the play.

> We shall define philosophy as total perspective, as mind
> overspreading life and forging chaos into unity.... Philosophy
> is harmonized knowledge making a harmonious life; it is the
> self-discipline which lifts us to serenity and freedom.
> Knowledge is power, but only wisdom is liberty.[3]

For most persons, the philosophy and principles of those who provide
agency leadership is of vital importance. These beliefs and values influence the priorities of agency goals and objectives; they influence the
performance and work satisfaction of every employee. They influence
the caliber of patient care and agency services.

These words may be simply a plethora of pious platitudes unless
translated into a program performance plan that includes all elements
that comprise the foundation for PONS.

Goals

A goal is a specific statement of purpose, an aim. What is the goal of
your unit? Has the goal been communicated to everyone on the unit?
Do employees understand the goal and relate it to the purpose of their
own jobs?

The goal of a patient care unit must necessarily relate to the goals of
the nursing department and the hospital. The primary purpose of the
hospital is to meet patient needs. This goal can be achieved most effectively only within a truly integrated hospital system. Such a system is
characterized by suitably differentiated activities and functional goals
of the specialized departments, but with one primary goal to which all
communication and interaction between departments is essential to
avoid goal-setting in isolation, and to assure that departmental goals
and objectives lead to effective fulfillment of the combined overall purpose of the organization. Indeed, as recognized in *Patient Care
Systems* by Kraegel, Mousseau, Goldsmith, and Arora, "A whole new,
orderly way of thinking about meeting patient needs has emerged. It
presses for a reorganization of resources in the healthcare field which
must be recognized. The hospital must be restructured for the patient.
This is the growing edge."[4]

Objectives

An objective is a specific task-oriented statement of results to be
achieved in order to accomplish a goal. Whereas a goal is a long-term

statement of purpose, an objective is a shorter-term statement of a specific target or aim. An objective presents a mutually developed and agreed-upon statement of who is going to do how much of what, how well, and when. The written objective can be clearly stated in a simple declarative sentence: "Somebody does something."

An extensive and detailed presentation of goals and objectives as related to patient care management is included in the chapter on Management by Objectives in Part III. The Objectives Worksheet described therein is helpful in problem solving, planning a mutually-agreed-upon course of action, reminding others of their expected participation, recording progress (one worksheet for each objective), assisting in developing a Program Performance Plan (PPP Schedule) for all objectives, evaluating results, and documenting action (for personnel file, accreditation and auditing purposes, legal evidence, and other reasons related to your management functions of planning-doing-controlling).

The Objectives Worksheet has been helpful to nurses and nurse managers in achieving objectives as diverse as (short term) changing an aide's pattern of arriving late for work, to (long term) implementing a two and a half year program performance plan for a family-centered maternal and child health service.

Definitions

Definitions, as used for this element of the foundation for PONS, refers to the act of making clear and distinct; a determining of outline, extent or limits. The process of developing meaningful definitions can be exciting, thought-provoking, challenging, and enlightening. Carefully and creatively carried out, it becomes a uniquely educative learning process. A dictionary is helpful—several copies, for expediting work in a group. The dictionary is necessary not for nit-picking, hairsplitting gameplaying, but for reasons of accuracy and precise usage. Professional people, regardless of title, are expected to set a professional example in the use of the simplest accurate words to convey meanings and facilitate understanding.

What needs defining? In the context of the foundation for PONS, the definitions have to do with the answers to such questions as: What's the nature of our business (occupation, concern, interest) on this unit? Whom do we serve? What is our source of patients? What type of care are we expected to provide (acute, long term, self, out-patient, home, etc.)? Who receives care (children, families, elderly, indigent, etc.)?

What do our patients (or clients) expect from us on this unit? To what extent do we expect patients (and/or their families) to participate in their own care? What is our relationship to other agency departments? What does patient care mean to us on this unit? What is the scope of nursing care? What is a patient need? What responsibilities do our unit personnel have to persons other than their nurse manager and patients? How are performance results evaluated?

These questions may suggest others that need answering in addition to or instead of the foregoing for your particular unit, department or agency. Do not be concerned if such questions seem to overlap with your goals and objectives. They should. They influence one another. Your exploration of such questions with others can lead to a set of definitions and statements that become part of your unit profile, a kind of self-developed charter expressing much that is fundamental to the functioning of your organizational unit and your principles of practice.

Function

A function is the natural or proper action for which a person, office, mechanism, or organ is fitted or employed; assigned duty or activity; specific occupation or role. The functions of the members of the nursing staff comprise another important building block in the foundation for PONS. One of the best ways for clarifying functions is the use of performance descriptions for every person in every job on your unit. Such performance descriptions are described in Chapter 1, and treated more fully in the ROPEP chapter of Part III.

Copies of performance descriptions for all unit personnel need to be available for review and use by every person. More effective team results occur when every person understands not only his own performance responsibilities but also what is expected of all the other team members too. We have previously noted that specialization and differentiation of functions, together with a unifying or integrating force, are necessary and desirable for the departments of an entire agency. The same principle applies at the unit level; differentiation of individual performance responsibilities, together with an effective integrating force, are necessary components for goal achievement.

Education

Education is the process of educating; the skills or knowledge so developed. Education has always been, and will continue to be, an essential and respected segment of the principles of nursing practice. Thus education is included as part of the foundation as well as being shown as a separate component. Its several aspects — inservice education, continuing education, and patient education — are discussed in Part IV.

Research

Research is scholarly or scientific investigation or inquiry. Research results are reported regularly in the pages of nursing publications. Increasingly, nurses in agency settings are carrying out research studies and scientific inquiries within their departments of nursing on a specific unit or units. In one notable VA Hospital, the innovative chief nurse stimulated her nurses to initiate a number of mini-research projects on subjects of their own choice. Typical study titles were as follows: How Close Are We to the Patients' Goals?, Evaluation of Patient Bathing, Inter-Disciplinary Analysis to Meeting Needs of Emphysema Patients, Study of Nursing Assistant Activities on a Single Unit, and Study of Unit Escort Service.

These mini-research projects were carried out by individual nurses, most of whom were previously overawed at the prospect of doing research. Guidance was provided in the use of the steps involved in a simple research design. The nurses did an excellent job of presenting oral and written project reports which included: Statement of Purpose, Methodology, Findings, Conclusions, Recommendations. The process of preparing for, carrying out, and reporting upon these mini-research projects generated much pride, esprit de corps, and useful results. Many recommendations were implemented. This kind of activity at the patient care unit level deserves to be emulated by other nurse managers. It enriches the foundation for PONS.

One form of research is literature research. This is, in effect, researching the research results of others. It involves a systematic inquiry into the investigations of others who have studied one or more facets of the subject in which you are interested. A classic example of this kind of research is the scholarly work by Herzberg, Mausner, Peterson, and Capwell at Psychological Service of Pittsburgh in which they reviewed almost two thousand writings to classify problem areas of job attitudes.[5] As part of their 279-page publication, Herzberg et al. present results from 15 studies including over 28,000 employees that identify factors contributing to either satisfaction or dissatisfaction. In his continuing work and writings, Herzberg concluded that the job factors influencing satisfaction could be grouped in two main classifications—the hygiene factors (affecting job dissatisfaction) and the motivators (affecting job satisfaction). His further work led to his familiar and popularized concepts of job enrichment and motivation through the work itself.[6] Nurses who wish to do so can initiate their own research. It might involve simply literature review in a specific subject area. Or your research might include a limited on-the-job scientific investigation of a specific hypothesis (an assumption subject to verification or proof). For example, after becoming sufficiently familiar with PONS, you may wish to test the following hypothesis (or some limited portion of it): the problem-oriented system leads to better patient care than a nonproblem-oriented system ("better patient care" being defined as a higher level of accomplishment in meeting patient needs).

Then, following some easy-to-understand guidelines, you can observe and evaluate two sets of patients—one group cared for using all of the components of PONS, the other group cared for without using the defined data base, the problem list, the numbered and titled care plans, or the SOAP-oriented progress notes. Your findings and conclusions could become a valuable contribution to your associates and your patients. At the very least, it would be an exciting learning experience for yourself and your unit associates.

The six building blocks—goals, definitions, objectives, functions, education, research—together with the underlying philosophy, provide a firm, supportive base for a problem-oriented nursing system. Such a solid foundation permits the nursing process to be utilized in ways that provide great satisfaction to the nursing and medical staffs while effectively meeting patient needs.

THE NURSING PROCESS AND PONS

The nursing process was discussed in Chapter 1 in connection with the management process and Figure 1:1. Mention was made of the fact that too often nurses themselves do not comprehend or use the nursing process in any significant way. But when the nursing process is understood as a component of PONS within the framework of the patient care process as depicted in Table 2:1, it acquires renewed meaning and utility. Our purpose now is to review the nursing process as an essential component of a problem oriented system.

The nursing process includes four phases: assessing, planning, implementing, evaluating. Yura and Walsh provide this definition: "The nursing process is an orderly, systematic manner of determining the client's problems, making plans to solve them, initiating the plan or assigning others to implement it, and evaluating the extent to which the plan was effective in resolving the problems identified."[7] According to Combs, the helping process must be as predictable as the helpers can make it.[8] When the helper is a nurse, she has a tool at her command—in the very nature of the nursing process—which becomes a facilitator of predictability. This process of improving predictability begins with the assessment of the person who becomes a patient. "Assess" means to appraise; estimate; form a tentative opinion; form a judgement of worth or significance. It also means to evaluate. In colloquial terms assess means to size up a situation, a person, or a patient's condition. Assessment leads to identification of the patient's problems and needs.

Assessment in the nursing process begins when the nurse takes a nursing history, by whatever name. This may be recorded on the nursing data base, patient profile, patient history, or initial nursing assessment. It involves communication, observation and perception. This is a time when needs, problems and some tentative goals are being expressed and identified by both patient and nurse. In some instances the family or significant others may be the only persons able to help with this initial patient assessment.

"Plan" means to formulate a program for the accomplishment or attainment of a goal. Once an assessment of needs and problems has been made, planning begins. Planning, insofar as possible, should be done with the patient and family rather than for them. Goals can be developed, and initial objectives identified, for each need or problem.

Setting patient care objectives is an integral part of the planning phase of the nursing process. The initial objectives are those that are developed upon admission of the patient. As needs change and new problems arise and are assessed, then plans—including objectives—will change too. Since these objectives are intended to be stated as part of the nursing plan, it is not necessary to create yet another nursing form for them. You may want to revise existing forms to assure that the nursing care plans are a part of the patient's permanent medical record.

As you carry out the planning phase of the nursing process, remember that you as a nurse can and must mutually set as many goals and objectives as possible with the patient and family. By so doing, you will be acting consistently within the foundation for PONS, and laying the groundwork for a successful discharge plan.

"Implement" is defined as a means employed to achieve a given end; to initiate and complete the actions necessary to accomplish an objective. Implementing implies doing, taking action. The successful achievement of an objective necessitates taking action. The action may involve several steps or just one or two. (The application of the management-by-objectives technique in nursing is presented in Part III.) For example, consider the situation of Mrs. Alexander who is recovering from a cerebral vascular accident which paralyzed her right side. Jane Doe, Mrs. Alexander's primary nurse, identifies the necessary goal as increasing the range of motion of Mrs. Alexander's right arm as much as possible. To achieve this goal, Jane has as one of her objectives to help Mrs. Alexander achieve the following: exercises right arm by herself at least four times a day. Possible steps to achieve this objective might include:

1. Discussing the whole idea of exercising with Mrs. Alexander, including how and why to exercise her arm by herself and her feelings about it (as reinforcement for instruction by the physical therapist.)
2. Setting an objective mutually with Mrs. Alexander, for exercising her right arm.
3. Making suitable entry on the nursing care plan.
4. Beginning the exercises by demonstrating how to do it with the use of her good left arm and hand.
5. Allowing Mrs. Alexander to return the demonstration, assisting her only as necessary.
6. Giving encouragement and praise as appropriate.
7. Having Mrs. Alexander do the exercising on her own schedule and without assistance.
8. Carefully recording Mrs. Alexander's progress in her patient record, using a patient teaching flow sheet.

The implementation phase of the nursing process is the one within which nurses can really make a significant change in the delivery of healthcare. It is at this point—while carrying out the care plan—that nurses can shift their emphasis from performing daily routine chores to a goal-oriented focus on meeting individual patient needs and helping to resolve individual patient problems. In the case of Mrs. Alexander's objective, the purpose is not simply to "get Mrs. Alexander to exercise her arm," but rather to help her understand the need for progressively increasing her range of arm motion so that she continually prevents contractures or muscle atrophy in her paralyzed arm. Having a daily objective in terms of achieving a specified degree range of motion helps Mrs. Alexander's motivation and sense of progress.

The conscious, deliberate and careful attention to mutual objectives in the implementation phase is the responsibility of nurses, working with their patients.

"Evaluate" means to examine and judge; to ascertain the value of; to appraise. Implicit in the evaluation phase of the nursing process is taking a look at the results of the nursing actions to see how well the nurse, patient and family have met the objectives (and ultimately the goals) they have established. Thus, at the time of Mrs. Alexander's discharge from the hospital, the nurse's discharge summary will include a notation such as: "Has achieved a 75° range of motion in right arm using lifting exercises which she can do herself unassisted, four times a day. Mrs. Alexander says, 'I know I have to continue these exercises every day in order to achieve my goal of greater range of motion of my right arm.'"

The nurse, as a key member of the helping professions, is in a uniquely advantageous position to lead and coordinate team efforts in meeting patient needs. Skillful use of the nursing process, as an essential component of PONS, will continue to be necessary. The process will be enhanced when the nurse recognizes and effectively utilizes both the technical mode and the human mode in getting results. We will see now how the problem-oriented record simplifies and adds a whole new dimension to the nursing process—and to the opportunities and satisfactions of being a nurse.

THE PROBLEM-ORIENTED RECORD

A problem-oriented record is a written account of events and facts related to identified and numbered problems of a person who has become a patient. The problem-oriented record is a particular kind of documentation for the patient's chart, the medical record kept for each patient. When only nursing personnel are involved in using the charting method unique to the problem-oriented system, then that portion of the patient's record is defined as a problem-oriented nursing record. Components of the problem-oriented nursing record are (1) a nursing data base, (2) a problem list, (3) a nursing plan and (4) the nursing progress notes.

Each component needs to be understood and used appropriately if the problem-oriented nursing record is to have real meaning for the patient. And this is what the record is all about; namely, a better means to help in meeting the needs of a person who has assumed the role of patient. The events and facts alluded to in the definition of a problem-oriented record are very real happenings for the person involved. They are truly vital statistics, events and facts. As such, they must be recorded accurately and legibly in all details: dates and times of events and facts; signatures (initials alone are not acceptable) and titles of nursing personnel; quotation marks around statements made by patient, family and significant others; concise statements of observations made by nursing personnel; notation of quantities and other relevant statistics. We present now each component of the problem-oriented nursing record.

Nursing Data Base

The nursing record begins when a person enters a healthcare agency for care. The agency may be a public health clinic, a mental health center, a general hospital, a state mental hospital or any one of a number of kinds of specialized hospitals, clinics or centers. Whatever the setting, basic information about the patient is required to help nursing personnel identify patient needs and problems. A variety of titles are used to identify the patient's data base. Some of these are nursing data base, nursing patient profile, nursing admission history, nursing assessment sheet, nursing history and nursing interview. Regardless of title, these records provide data that serves as a base line, the basic starting point for measurement and comparison purposes.

The information contained in a nursing data base is obtained by the nurse in the initial assessment phase of the nursing process. Assessment requires proficiency in interviewing and observing. A nurse learns proficiency in these techniques by using the necessary skills, by practicing the right method and using it repeatedly. A skill, remember, is proficiency in a way of doing something using one's hands, body and brain. During the process of interviewing, the nurse is also observing the patient for behaviors, mannerisms, physical signs and symptoms, physical expression of feelings. Practice of the necessary skills will help to sharpen observing ability. When skillful interviewing is combined with skillful observing, the assessment process is most likely to yield a meaningful patient data base. Accurate observation depends on the skill of the nurse and the nature of the observation criteria.

Problem List

A problem is anything that causes concern to the patient and his family or to the nursing staff and others concerned with the patient's care. Walker et al. define a problem as "anything that requires diagnosis or management or that interferes with the quality of life as perceived by the patient."[9]

The problem list derives from the data base. It is advisable and desirable to have a complete list of all the patient's problems, such as would be available when a problem-oriented medical record is in use. In any event it is necessary to identify pertinent problems as the patient presents them. The problem list, however, is not fixed and unchanging. The number of problems will increase as new problems are identified and will change as some problems are resolved.

When a problem-oriented medical record is in use, the problem list is usually located at the front of the patient's record for ready reference. When only a problem-oriented nursing record is being used, the problem list may be located at the front of the nursing section of the patient's record as a single sheet. Or the problem list may be combined with nursing orders, actions or directives— which constitute the nursing care plan.

The use of the subscript "n" with the problem number is a means of coping with the following question. "If the medical staff adopts a problem-oriented medical record at some later time, will confusion occur in use of problem numbers in older patient records where only nurses assign numbers?" One way to avoid any possibility of such confusion is for nursing personnel to use the subscript "n" with each problem number. This identifies it for all time as a problem number assigned by nursing. Later when the medical staff adopts POMR, the "n" subscript no longer is needed since both nurses and doctors will then use the same problem list and numbers.

When many problems have been identified, it is useful and time-saving to refer to the problem by both its number and name rather than using just the number alone. (ie: Problem $\#2_n$—Nausea and Vomiting). Remember that the nurse does not determine medical diagnosis. Once the doctor has made a diagnosis, however, the nurse should include it on the nursing problem list. The following list, Identifying and Classifying Problems, provides some problem categories and examples of specific evidence of such problems.

Each problem is numbered consecutively beginning with one. Once a problem has been given a number, the two become inseparable; the number is not assigned to any other problem, even when the prior problem is resolved. One good reason for this is that the problem may recur. If it does, the same number is there ready to be used, thereby avoiding confusion. Another reason is that the same number is always used to identify the same problem on the nursing care plan, the progress notes and wherever else that problem is referred to in nursing documentation. So each plan of action, each nursing directive, each progress note is done in terms of a specific problem rather than at random.

IDENTIFYING AND CLASSIFYING PROBLEMS

Categories	*Examples*
Medical problems	
A diagnosis	Myocardial Infarction
Signs or Symptoms	Shortness of breath
Abnormal laboratory findings	Abnormal EKG
Surgical problems	
An operation	Myocardial Revascularization
Psychological problems	
Psychiatric	Suicidal
Behavioral	Defensive
Sociological problems	
	Loss of income
	Marital friction
Demographic problems	
	Farmer for 20 years; now unable to farm
Other problems (active/inactive)	
An allergy	Morphine
An operation	Appendectomy
A risk factor	Overweight

An Asset List

Dr. W. P. Mazur describes a most useful innovation in his adaptation of the problem-oriented system.[10] He and his staff at Osawatomie State Hospital in Kansas have developed a separate form for a listing of each patient's assets, which are whatever may be identified as special attributes and strengths of a patient and his life situation that may be marshalled to assist in his care planning, and facilitate his return to normal health and daily functioning. These may include attitudes, habits, beliefs; special skills, talents, hobbies; resources, facilities, and support available from family members and/or the community.

Dr. Mazur suggests listing patient assets in order of availability (how rapidly can they be used?), magnitude or intensity (most outstanding, strongest), and location (intrapersonal, interpersonal, community). A letter-coding of assets (A, B, C, in contrast to the number-coded problem list) makes possible ready cross reference in the nursing data base, care plans, progress notes, discharge plans or other records. An asset list has special applicability in psychiatric hospitals and other long-term care facilities. Partly because of our firm belief in the necessity for building on assets, we see significant benefits in the use of the asset list as part of PONS in other agencies too.

The Nursing Care Plan

The nursing care plan is the document which clearly states the patient's problems, together with the objectives, methods and strategies for resolving the patient's problems and needs. The medical plan of care is written as the doctor's orders with each order dated, signed and carried out in strict adherance to the instructions. The nursing plan of care needs to be handled in a similar fashion, with each nurse's order (instruction or directive) dated, signed and carried out by the nursing staff with the same degree of thoroughness as with the doctors' orders. Doctors' orders are not written in pencil, unsigned, on a Kardex which is erased and discarded upon discharge of the patient. Nurses' orders must no longer be so treated. They, as well as the doctors' orders, must become a permanent part of the patient's chart. Unless and until the nursing care plan is accorded the importance it deserves there is little likelihood of its being taken seriously by members of the nursing staff. Written policies, procedures, and consistent management follow through are required to lend meaning and support to the nursing plan of care.

The nursing care plan is intended to be flexible, to change as the patient's needs and problems change. It is important that planning, as evidenced by the nursing care plan, become an integral part of the patient's record. It must not be erased, written over, or discarded. Some interesting ways to achieve this are being utilized in a variety of healthcare settings. It is not essential to use a separate card (such as Kardex) for the care plan. What is essential is that the plan meet the criteria set forth in the following list:

Criteria For The Nursing Care Plan

The nursing care plan:

1. Is initiated on the date of admission.
2. Is in writing as a part of the patient's permanent record.
3. Is based on identification of specific problems and needs of the patient.
4. Is coordinated with the medical care plan.
5. Is based upon scientific principles and is therapeutically effective.
6. Insures maximum physical and emotional safety and security for the patient.
7. Reflects immediate and long-range planning for regaining or maintaining maximum degree of health attainable for the patient.
8. Identifies and meets the psychosocial and physiological needs of the patient.
9. Provides for patient and family participation as much as possible.
10. Includes patient and family teaching/learning programs and discharge planning.
11. Indicates specific nursing care measures to be taken.
12. Specifies objectives, methods and approaches to assure best results for patient.
13. Is contributed to and used by all nursing personnel involved in the care of the patient.

A useful exercise for many readers will be to use the nursing care plan criteria as follows. First select the nursing records for five of your present patients. From these records, identify how well the specific nursing care plans meet the criteria as listed. This simple exercise can be most revealing. You may find more evidence of complete, documented planning than you expected. Or you may find very little such evidence. In effect, you have been performing a nursing mini-audit.

Secondly, review the forms you are now using for their adequacy in filling your needs. Can you create new forms that you think would be more useful than the ones you are using? Remember that the forms you design and use are a means to the end of meeting the criteria for nursing care plans — and thus optimizing patient care. Thirdly, suggest some ways you might meet some of the other criteria as listed.

The total process of planning requires the cooperation of both medical and nursing staffs with the administration of the hospital. The nurse can prove to be of invaluable service to the patient if he/she looks upon the patient first as a person, then as a patient, and then as a part of a planning process. The patient must become a part of the planning process. It is, after all, his illness. No one is more concerned with it than he is, even when his family and significant others show similar concern.

The written nursing care plan is intended to be a practical plan of action that individualizes the care of a patient and makes possible meaningful continuity of care. The planning process begins with assessment via the nursing history, interview of the patient, and the medical history. The plan should be based on specific goals of the patient, as well as those of the nurse and physician, and should be flexible. It will change, perhaps daily or hourly, as the patient changes. It becomes a permanent part of the patient's record and is used in any referrals that are made for the patient upon discharge.

Nursing Progress Notes

Once an initial plan of action has been determined for the patient, the implementation of that plan begins. The Joint Commission on Accreditation of Hospitals (JCAH) indicates in its standards that the care provided shall be safe, efficient and therapeutically effective; and shall be documented. Specifically, JCAH states: "Nursing records and reports that reflect the patient's progress, and the nursing care planned, must be maintained. These records and reports should demonstrate adherence to the objectives of the nursing service. To contribute to continuity of patient care, the nursing notes on the patient's medical record should be significant, accurate and concise."[11]

The problem-oriented nursing record provides for the concise, accurate recording of significant information about the patient and his care through the use of (1) the SOAP format on the nursing progress notes; (2) a discharge summary, and (3) the use of flow sheets for repetitive components of care.

The Soap Format

Problem #:   Problem Name:
S: Subjective information: Includes what the patient says. Use quotation marks; or note that patient stated something, and what he communicated.

O: Objective information: First-hand observations made by nursing personnel.

A: Assessment: Based on subjective and objective information. This is the conclusion the nurse makes.

P: Plan of action.

The use of the SOAP format requires ability in communication, especially listening and observing; skill in the analysis of data; knowledge of clinical information and appropriate terminology; planning and organizing of information; and appropriate action. Learning the skills requires practice and patience. Some nurses question the need for using all of the four SOAP components all of the time. Common sense, observed practice and judgment indicate the need for including all four steps all of the time. However, the entry for one or another of the SOAP items may be simply "none," "no change," or a dash to indicate no new data available. Mazur provides in his manual *The Problem-Oriented System in The Psychiatric Hospital* some of the best examples of the flexibility of the SOAP format, as well as some examples of SOA, OAP, and SAP notes.[12]

Flow Sheets

Flow sheets provide an efficient and time-saving way to record information that must be obtained repeatedly at regular and/or short intervals of time. Usually such necessary information, accumulated without suitable flow sheets, clutters the progress notes and defeats the purpose of the SOAP format. The nursing care flow sheet does not substitute for progress notes, but is used to supplement them.

Flow sheets can be used to record information on such things as vital signs, intake and output, treatments, post-operative care, post partum care and diabetic regimen—to mention only a few. The rule of thumb is to use a flow sheet whenever information needs to be documented repeatedly, and can be done adequately by numbers or check marks.

Discharge Summary

The nursing discharge summary is more than the conventional recording of the date, time and mode by which the patient leaves a healthcare facility—as pertinent as these may be upon the occasion of actual discharge. The nursing discharge summary is the direct result of planning for discharge that begins soon after the person becomes a patient and is admitted to a healthcare agency. Evidence of discharge planning should be documented throughout the patient's stay. It should be in evidence and recognized by the patient and his family. It should be retrievable from the documentation in the nursing care plan, the progress notes and flow sheets.

The actual discharge summary of a patient should include: (1) his state of health now compared with his state at the time of admission; (2) his activity level; (3) his knowledge and feelings about his state of health, medications, diet, activity, equipment and supplies, referral, follow-up care and resources available in the community. Patients, upon discharge, require information that is highly specific to them. The kind, amount and detail of the information depends upon each patient's own unique needs in a given situation. It also depends on other variables such as the person's knowledge, feelings, values, prejudices, life style and experiences in living and working, as well as the amount and kind of intrusions upon his health status. Patient teaching, based upon these variables and on standards of care for specific illnesses, helps each individual to learn what he or she needs to know at the time of discharge. The discharge summary is intended as a final entry by the nurse in the patient's record. It may be a part of the progress notes, or it may be a more extensive summary on a separate form.

Discharge planning requires a collaborative effort on the part of all members of a healthcare team. Doctors, nurses, therapists, nutritionists, and many others may need to pool their efforts to provide good continuity of care from one healthcare setting to another and into the patient's home. The nurse can and should play a pivotal role in coordinating the efforts of all those involved, including the patient and his family. Since the discharge summary is prepared on the patient's behalf, each patient should receive a copy of his discharge summary.

In Summary

The problem-oriented nursing record offers nurses the particular opportunity to integrate the care they give with a way of documenting that care. We know that for nurses accustomed to traditional practices much time and effort is required to change long-standing habit patterns. But we also believe that the effort is worth it. Nurses cannot rely upon sketchy notes supplemented by memory and share it all verbally. The complexity of healthcare today no longer encourages or permits such practices. They are neither safe nor efficient. Random-style charting and traditional narrative notes fall into the same category.

The problem-oriented record as part of an entire problem-oriented system is no panacea — but it has been well tested; it works well; it holds great continuing promise for patients and for nurses. We believe strongly that nurses generally can and will bring that promise into full realization.

THE NURSING AUDIT AND PONS

Nursing audit is the fourth component of the problem-oriented nursing system. Audit plays an essential role in the system. It is the inspection function. It is part of the quality assurance program. Not only is it essential; it is mandatory for JCAH accreditation. Nursing audit is defined as a method for assuring documentation of the quality of nursing care in keeping with the standards of the agency, the nursing department, and the professional, governmental and accrediting groups.

Among those who are concerned with quality control in industry, there is a familiar statement that rings true: "You cannot inspect quality into a product; quality must be built into the product or service." So it is in nursing and the other helping relationships within healthcare agencies. The level of quality is determined at the point of service. People provide service to and for patients. People determine the quality level of the care being provided. This level of care, however it is experienced and perceived by the patient, may or may not be so reflected in the audit results. Part of the reason for PONS is to assure that patient needs are met with an appropriate level of care which is reflected accurately in the audit reports.

Too often in the past the patient's record has not reflected, accurately and completely, the excellence of the nursing care actually provided to the patient. Nursing care plans maintained conscientiously from day to day in the open chart, have (in some hospitals) been removed and destroyed by nursing service as a regular practice when the patient was discharged. This action effectively eliminated from the closed chart vital evidence of the quality of nursing care provided to the patient. An organized audit procedure will lead to corrective action in such cases, and assure preservation of the necessary data in an appropriate way.

Here are the major purposes and benefits of a systematic nursing audit procedure. Nursing audit:

1. Necessitates adequate documentation of the nursing care provided to the patient through the entire nursing process.
2. Directs attention to the design and utility of the charting records.
3. Encourages use of the Problem-Oriented Nursing System.
4. Supports, and becomes an integral part of, the Nursing by Objectives Program.
5. Facilitates the cooperative planning and delivery of patient care by physicians and nursing personnel.
6. Increases the priority for a Results-Oriented Performance Evaluation Program for nursing service employees.
7. Enriches and provides direction to inservice education efforts.
8. Provides a specific management technique to aid nurse managers in carrying out their evaluation and control function.
9. Identifies ways to improve patient care, both short range and long range.
10. Provides a meaningful way for nursing staff members to participate and achieve career growth.

Nursing Audit and the Problem-Oriented Nursing Record (PONR)

Nursing audit, like any other management technique, works best when it is used as part of an integrated system. Before beginning an audit program, it is worthwhile to examine the components of the patient care system within which nursing audit is to be introduced in the specific healthcare agency. In order to do this, it is helpful to have a frame of reference from which to begin. The problem-oriented nursing system, inclusive of the nursing process, provides such a frame of reference.

The audit procedure is an aspect of the evaluation phase of the ongoing nursing process. Implementation of the audit procedure is greatly facilitated when a problem-oriented charting system is used. The very nature and purpose of problem-oriented charting is to provide for reliable evaluation of a patient's problems, progress and treatment results. A more complete presentation of nursing audit as a nursing management technique is provided in Part III.

As a management technique, nursing audit is part of the evaluating and planning phases of the management process. It is ongoing rather than sporadic. Monthly and quarterly comparisons of results provide a way to determine the efficacy of the audit program.

The retrospective audit procedure may focus on either an outcome audit or a process audit. The outcome audit identifies patient outcomes that are unsatisfactory, and is intended to identify also the patterns of nursing care that appear to be responsible. The process audit is a deeper probe of already recognized (or suspected) problems in the nursing care process.

In Summary

Nursing care quality is becoming more measureable and quantifiable. It can be and is being translated into numbers. While this trend may not be easy for some nurses to accept or comprehend, for other nurses it is most welcome. Experience in every field of human endeavor indicates that when quality or performance standards are established and results are measured against such standards, then the results improve. There is every reason to believe that this ongoing process in patient care will contribute to greater, not less, satisfaction among nursing personnel within their chosen profession.

Nursing audit is a major vital component of PONS, a patient-centered system with:

- the problem-oriented record as a central data repository and control;
- the nursing process as the coordinating, integrating force modelled on the scientific method;
- nursing audit and education as the two companion measuring/correcting mechanisms, maintaining the feedback and revision functions;
- the foundation as the soundly-structured supportive base for the dynamic, producing system for meeting patient needs;

- the whole system friction-proofed with the lubricant of a modern blend of technical and human modes for the helpers who make it work.

NOTES

1. Edith P. Lewis, "The Care of the Sick, *"Nursing Outlook*, 22 (October 1974), p. 625.

2. For historical background, see W.T. Mazur, *The Problem-Oriented System in the Psychiatric Hospital* (Garden Grove, Calif.: Trainex Press, 1974), pp. 7-9.

3. Will Durant, *The Mansions of Philosophy*, (Garden City, N.Y.: Garden City Pub. Co., 1929), pp. viii, ix,x. (Newer publication available by the title *The Pleasures of Philosophy*, published by Simon & Schuster, 1953). Reprinted with permission of Simon & Schuster, Inc., © 1953.

4. Janet Kraegel et al, *Patient Care Systems* (Philadelphia: J.B. Lippincott, 1974), p.viii.

5. Frederick Herzberg et al, *Job Attitudes: Review of Research and Opinion* (Pittsburgh: Psychological Service of Pittsburgh, 1957).

6. Idem. "One more time: How do you motivate employees?" *Harvard Business Review*, 46 (January-February 1968), pp. 53-62.

7. Helen Yura and Mary Walsh, *The Nursing Process* (Washington Catholic University of America Press, 1967), p. 23.

8. A.W. Combs, D.L. Avila and W.W. Purkey, *Helping Relationships: Basic Concepts for the Helping Professions* (Boston: Allyn and Bacon, 1971) , p.166.

9. H. Kenneth Walker, MD, *"The Problem-Oriented Medical Record."* or *Applying the Problem-Oriented System*, edited by H. K. Walker, MD; J. W. Hurst, MD; and M.F. Woody, RN (New York: Medcom Press, 1973), p.14.

10. W.T. Mazur, *The Problem-Oriented System in the Psychiatric Hospital* (Garden Grove, Calif.: Trainex Press, 1974), pp. 6, 15-16.

11. Joint Commission on Accreditation of Hospitals, *Accreditation Manual for Hospitals* (Chicago: Joint Commission on Accreditation of Hosptials, 1976) p. 124.

12. W.P. Mazur, op. cit., p. 61-65.

SUGGESTED READINGS

Books

Cantor, Marjorie M. *The JCAH Standards* (Wakefield, Mass.: Contemporary Publishing Co., 1974).

Carter, J.H.; Hilliard, M.; Castles, M.R.; Stoll L. D. and Cowan, A. *Standards of Nursing Care: A Guide for Evaluation* 2nd ed., enlarged (New York: Springer Publishing Co., 1976).

Easton, Richard. *Problem-Oriented Medical Record Concepts* (New York: Appleton-Century-Crofts, 1974).

Enslow, A. and Swisher, S. *Interviewing and Patient Care* (New York: Oxford University Press, 1972).

Epstein, Charlotte. *Effective Interaction in Contemporary Nursing* (Englewood Cliffs, N.J.: Prentice-Hall, Inc., 1974).

Froebe, D.J., RN, PhD. and Bain, K.J., RN, EdD. *Quality Assurance Programs and Controls in Nursing* (St. Louis: C.V. Mosby, 1976).

Futtrell, M. and Kelleher, M. *The Nurse's Guide to Health Services for Patients* (Boston: Little, Brown & Co., 1973).

Ganong, Joan and Warren. *HELP with the Problem-Oriented Nursing System* (Chapel Hill, N.C.: W.L. Ganong Co., 1975).

Gorton, John. *Behavioral Components of Patient Care* (New York: MacMillan, Inc., 1970).

Mayers, Marlene. *A Systematic Approach to the Nursing Care Plan* (New York: Appleton-Century-Crofts, 1972).

Mayers, Marlene. *Standard Nursing Care Plans* (Palo Alto, Calif.: R/P Co., Medical Systems, 1974 and 1975).

Mazur, W.P., MD. *The Problem-Oriented System in the Psychiatric Hospital* (Garden Grove, Cal.: Trainex Press, 1974).

Neelon, F.A., MD, and Ellis, G.J., MD. *A Syllabus of Problem-Oriented Patient Care* (Boston: Little, Brown & Co., 1974).

Phaneuf, M.C. *The Nursing Audit: Profile for Excellence* (New York: Appleton-Century-Crofts, 1972).

Nursing Clinics of North America. I. *The Problem-Oriented Record.* II. *Quality Assurance* (Philadelphia: W.B. Saunders Co., 1974).

Riehl, J. and Ray, C. *Conceptual Models for Nursing Practice.* (New York: Appleton-Century-Crofts, 1974).

Sherman, J. and Fields, S. *Guide to Patient Evaluation* (New York: Medical Examination Publishing Co., 1974).

Vasey, E. and Riley, M. *Quality Assurance: Peer Review for Nursing* (Pittsburgh: Western Pennsylvania Regional Medical Program, 1975).

Walker, H.K., MD; Hurst, J.W., MD; and Woody, M.F., RN, eds. *Applying the Problem-Oriented System* (New York: Medcom Press, 1973).

Weed, L.L. *Medical Records, Medical Education, and Patient Care* (New York: Appleton-Century-Crofts, 1972).

Weed, L.L. *Your Health Care and How to Manage It* (Burlington, Vt.: Promis Laboratory, 1975).

Wooley, F.R.; Warnick, M.W.; Kane, R.L.; and Dyer, Elaine D. *Problem-Oriented Nursing* (New York: Springer Publishing Co., 1974).

Yura, H. and Walsh, M. *The Nursing Process* (Washington, D.C.: The Catholic University of America Press, 1967).

Joint Commission on Accreditation of Hospitals. *Accreditation Manual for Hospitals* (Chicago: Joint Commission on Accreditation of Hospitals, 1973).

Articles

Lewis, Edith P., "The Care of the Sick," (Editorial), *Nursing Outlook*, 22 (October 1974), p. 625.

Tapia, Jayne, "The Nursing Process in Family Health," *Nursing Outlook*, 20 (April 1972).

Part III

Operational Management

Chapter 3
Management By Objectives

Setting goals and objectives in human endeavor is not new. From time immemorial farmers have set daily and yearly goals for themselves in terms of size and quality of crops. Seafarers have set trip goals and daily objectives, and measured their performance accordingly. Salesmen have traditionally set (or had set for them) sales quotas and been rewarded for exceeding those quotas.

Task-oriented quality and quantity standards for all kinds of work have been used commonly for measuring performance results. Organizationally, the amount of profits (and/or the quality of services) have been accepted as performance measures.

Only in fairly recent times, however, has there been a meaningful productive effort to develop and implement a system of performance objectives and standards especially for managers in our organizations and institutions. In 1954 Peter Drucker's management classic *The Practice of Management* first coined the term "management by objectives." Drucker wrote:

What business enterprise needs is a principle of management that will give full scope to individual strength and responsibility, as well as common direction to vision and effort, establish team work, and harmonize the goals of the individual with the commonweal. Management by objectives and self-control makes the commonweal the aim of every manager. It substitutes for control from outside the stricter, more exacting, and more effective control from inside. It motivates the manager to action, not because somebody tells him to do something or talks him into doing it, but because the objective task demands it. He acts not because somebody

wants him to but because he himself decides that he has to —
he acts, in other words, as a free man.

I do not use the word "philosophy" lightly; indeed I prefer
not to use it at all; it's much too big a word. But management
by objectives and self-control may properly be called a
philosophy of management. It rests on an analysis of the
specific needs of the management group and the obstacles it
faces. It rests on a concept of human action, behavior, and
motivation. Finally, it applies to every manager, whatever his
level and function, and to any organization whether large or
small. It insures performance by converting objective needs
into personal goals. And this is genuine freedom.[1]

During the fourth and fifth decades of this century, great progress
was made in the behavioral sciences. The names of many persons
who contributed to this progress became familiar to managers
everywhere — names such as Argyris, Bakke, Bennis, Brown, Drucker,
Etzioni, Gellerman, Herzberg, Jourard, Lewin, Likert, Maslow, Mayo,
McClelland, McGregor, Myers, Perls, Rogers. The prodigious output of
these researchers, teachers, and writers was combined with the great
work of earlier management consultants and practitioners, such as
Barnard, Fayol, Follett, Gantt, Gilbreth, Roethlisberger, Taylor, Ur-
wick, Wiener. MBO was one outgrowth of this evolution of theory,
thought, research and practice.

UNDERLYING CONCEPTS AND PHILOSOPHY

Marie DiVincenti, a director of nursing service, presents an excellent overview of management by objectives (MBO) and its relationship to other aspects of nurse management, including the need for administrative support. "Providing a supportive enviroment assures a
maximum probability that each staff member, in the light of his
background, values, desires, and expectations, will view each experience and interaction as supportive — as something which builds
and maintains his sense of personal worth and importance."[2] Yes, it is
important that a supportive enviroment exist for MBO to help every
employee satisfy his personal needs and goals and to help the entire
staff meet the immediate needs and objectives of the people who come
to them as patients and clients.

Since MBO is an outgrowth of the historical developments described
earlier in this chapter, it is a technique that is based upon some of the

findings about people that reflect a different view of the nature of man from the views commonly held by many managers in years past — and still retained by some. Theory X and Theory Y, as propounded by McGregor,[3] show the contrast between the assumptions and propositions about people that appear to be believed by old-school managers compared with research findings about the real nature of people (See Table 3:1).

Simplified for purposes of comparison, Theory X represents the view that people require authoritarian direction and control by managers to achieve organizational goals. Theory Y supports the view that the true nature of people is such that, with managerial leadership

---

Table 3:1
Comparison of Theories X and Y

ASSUMPTIONS AND PROPOSITIONS	THEORY X (Direction & Control)	THEORY Y (Participation & Self Control)
1. Management is responsible for organizing the elements of productive enterprise—money, materials, equipment, people—in the interest of economic ends.	Yes	Yes
2. With respect to people, this is a process of directing their efforts, motivating them, controlling their actions, modifying their behavior to fit the needs of the organization.	Yes	Yes—but with an enlightened interpretation of what these words mean.
3. The average man has an inherent dislike of work and avoids it if he can.	Yes	No—Physical and mental effort is as natural as play or rest.
4. He lacks ambition, dislikes responsibility, prefers to be led.	Yes	No—The evidence of these are generally the consequences of experience, not inherent human characteristics.
5. He is inherently self-centered, indifferent to organizational needs.	Yes	No—He is concerned with organizational needs when they can be identified with his own needs.
6. He is by nature resistant to change.	Yes	No—He may have learned to appear this way for reasons of self-protection.
7. He is gullible, not very bright, the ready dupe of the charlatan and the demagogue.	Yes	No—Imagination, ingenuity, and creativity are capacities which are widely, not narrowly distributed in the population.
8. People must be coerced, controlled, directed, threatened with punishment to get them to put forth adequate effort toward the achievement of organizational objectives.	Yes	No—These are not the only means for bringing about effort toward organizational objectives. Man will exercise self-direction and self-control in the service of objectives to which he is committed.

Adapted from Douglas McGregor, <u>The Human Side of Enterprise</u> (New York: McGraw-Hill, 1960).

that permits a high degree of involvement and participation, employees will direct their own efforts toward organizational goals as a means of meeting their own needs and objectives. Here is the message of Theory Y in its positive assumptions and propositions about people:

1. Physical and mental effort is as natural as play or rest.
2. Ambition and acceptance of responsibility are traits which come naturally to people. When they seem to be lacking, it is generally the consequence of experience.
3. People are concerned with, and will work toward accomplishing, organizational needs when they can be identified with their own needs.
4. People do not resist change; they resist being changed. People may have learned to appear resistant to change for reasons of self-protection.
5. Imagination, ingenuity and creativity are capacities which are widely distributed in the population.
6. People will exercise self-direction and self-control in the service of objectives to which they are committed.

ACHIEVING MUTUAL GOALS

The achievement of mutual goals is the anticipated outcome of management by objectives. People who work within the same organization usually have many similar goals. Nurse managers and nursing staff members serve as a case in point. One mutual goal held by both groups is the delivery of high quality care to patients. According to Douglas McGregor, mutual goal achievement requires a participative approach on the part of management acting on the "Y" assumptions about people. Management can arrange organizational conditions so that people can achieve their own goals by directing their efforts toward the goals of the organization within which they work. McGregor points out that this can be done best when management creates opportunities, releases potential, removes obstacles, encourages growth and provides necessary guidance. It is management by objectives rather than management by control.

The integration of hospital and nursing department goals with the needs and goals of individual nursing staff members — through mutual understanding, mutual trust, cooperative effort and leadership skill — can achieve meaningful results for all: the hospital administrator, the doctor, the nurse manager, the nursing staff members and the patients.

Dr. E. Wight Bakke in *Teamwork in Industry* pointed out that people want progress toward and security with respect to certain goals. The first of these is "the respect of their fellows," to be considered important and respectable by the people with whom they associate. Another goal Bakke refers to as "creature sufficiency," or the desire to have the amount of food, clothes, shelter, health which compares favorably with associates. People want "increasing control over their own affairs." They want their own decisions to be effective in shaping their lives, and to reduce the amount of control exercised by others over them. Bakke notes "understanding" as a goal. People want to know the score, to know the relation between what happens and what caused it to happen. They also want to be able to use the full range of their abilities, to have the chance to do the things they think they can do. Lastly, Bakke mentions "integrity" as a goal. This he describes as the desire of people to feel that their actions and principles are consistent, to feel that they are a significant part of the world about them.[4]

People working in healthcare settings have many similar goals regardless of their job titles. The goals referred to by Bakke can be identified among Maslow's hierarchy of five human needs. And we know that the unmet goals and needs serve as motivators for people. The nurse manager who understands the relationship between needs and self-motivation can use motivational methods and leadership techniques that lead to personal satisfaction of needs and goals while working in harmony with the goals of the organization. This is mutual goal setting at its best.

ACCOUNTABILITY AND CONTROL

The management process has control as one of its components. In the traditional approach to accountability described by McGregor, control systems have been used in which management sets performance standards and measures the results and then rewards employees who meet the standards and punishes those who fail to do so. The consequences of such a system may be identified as follows:

- The system works — but not as well as desired.
- There may be widespread antagonism to the controls and to those who administer them.
- Employees at all levels may offer successful resistance and non-

compliance to administrative controls.
- Performance information may well be unreliable due to the negative effect of resistance and noncompliance.
- There is a need for close surveillance of employees which dilutes delegation, impinges on the manager's time and impedes employee development.
- It creates high administrative costs.

Such an approach has a tendency to generate and accentuate noncompliance. When the pressure to comply is coupled with lack of trust and support the end result may be perceived as a threat. People often respond to threats through the use of defensive, hostile and protective behavior. A more productive approach to the control element of the management process is described by McGregor:

> When members of an organization are committed to the organization's goals, surveillance in the usual sense becomes largely unnecessary. The problem is not one of obtaining passive compliance but of enabling all parts of the organization to achieve the goals to which they are committed. Each unit down to the individual level has a degree of control over its own fate. The total process, from the initial exploration of reality to the solution of problems arising in the day-to-day attempt to meet goals and standards, provides ample opportunity for intrinsic rewards and for the motivational effects of intrinsic punishments arising from mistakes and failures.[5]

The nurse manager can apply a sound strategy that will assist with accountability and control. This strategy is based upon two principles: (1.) people's response to information about their performance varies with their commitment to goals, and (2.) to cope with reality requires open communication, mutual trust, mutual support and mutual working through of conflicts. The strategy includes the following steps:

1. An open presentation and discussion of the nurse manager's requirements for successful goal accomplishment at any given point in time; including review of external forces and internal problems shown by past performance.
2. A broad analysis of changes in performance required to meet the demands of reality.
3. An analysis of how everyone in the department can contribute

best to the organization effort — carried out face-to-face at all levels.

4. Statements from each patient unit of the goals and standards to which it commits itself. This includes an analysis of the help the unit feels is needed to accomplish the goals such as information feedback, staff resources, policy or procedure changes, and equipment and manpower needs.

The success of the strategy is dependent upon the intent and thoroughness with which it is used as well as the involvement of people at all levels. Properly implemented, this strategy leads to a type of self control and accountability consistent with a Theory Y philosophy.

These concepts and beliefs about people can be translated into daily productive action through appropriate use of management functions, techniques and skills. MBO is one such technique. The three basic steps of MBO (set objectives, perform, measure results) are, like the management functions, a cyclical process. Each phase builds upon the input from the one preceding. Each phase provides the feedback or output for the one that follows.

People who think together stay together. This paraphrase of a familiar slogan carries much meaning for those who use MBO. Much thinking together — using the variety of performance skills in communicating, conceptualizing, perceiving, discussing, problem solving, understanding, compromising, decision making — is desirable at the outset of an organization-wide MBO program. This is because goals and objectives at the departmental or unit level of a healthcare agency need to be related to the broader divisional and organizational goals and objectives. Staying together, literally and figuratively, is then possible. A sequential plan of action follows in Figure 3:1. (See also Appendix F for a pertinent example of the goals and annual objectives for Nebraska Methodist Hospital.)

THOUGHT PRECEDES ACTION

Combs et al. wrote in *Helping Relationships,* "a helper's conceptions of the goals he is seeking to accomplish have inexorable effects upon his behavior.... Goals and purposes determine action."[6] These words provide a useful transition from the concepts and philosophical considerations of the foregoing paragraphs to the pragmatic aspects of MBO in healthcare settings.

The steps in the Plan for MBO may appear to be a logical, necessary sequence of events leading from the translation of the purpose and

Figure 3:1
Plan For MBO

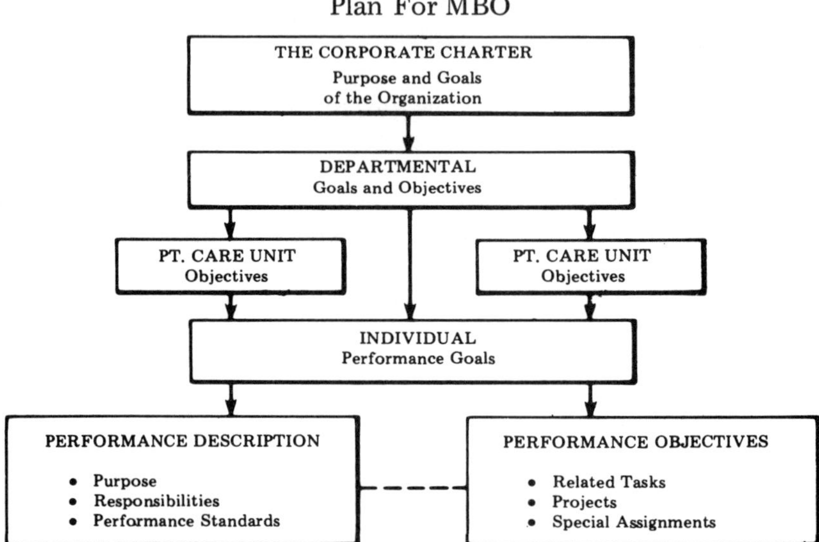

The Corporate Charter (Purpose of the Organization)

Every organization exists for some purpose. This is stated in the articles of incorporation. The purpose is often elaborated in the form of a number of specific goals with specific objectives identified annually.

Departmental Goals and Objectives

Each division, section, department and unit exists to help achieve the purpose of the organization. Thus departmental goals and objectives need to be identified in writing, consistent with the organizational purpose, but departmentally distinctive as related to the department's special function. Specific objectives for each patient care unit are essential.

Job Purpose, Responsibilities, and Objectives

Within each department, people work at jobs to help achieve departmental goals and objectives. Thus a performance description identifies for each person the purpose, responsibilities, and measures of satisfactory performance to be met.

Beyond the normal performance responsibilities, however, are related tasks, projects, and special assignments. These are the short or longer-term activities necessary to attain identified objectives that are steppingstones to goal achievement.

goals of the corporate organization (hospital, nursing home, school) to the development of departmental and unit goals and objectives, and thence to the development of the performance goals and objectives for individual employees. But too often the process does not work this way. Sometimes one or more of the initial steps are not carried out, or receive only cursory attention. What then? Can department heads, the nursing director, patient care coordinators, or head nurses still proceed to use MBO in their own areas? Yes! Sometimes, for identifiable reasons, the only way to begin is at the departmental or unit level. In such cases, the person initiating the program will certainly need to do so with the knowledge and approval of his or her own manager, using whatever broad statements are available, written or understood, of institution-wide and/or department-wide goals.

Assume that you plan to take the initiative to begin using MBO for your own area of responsibility, whatever your position title in your hospital. Insofar as you know (and you have inquired) there are no available written statements of the goals and objectives of the larger organizational unit (such as maternal and child care, nursing service department, or the entire hospital) of which you and your co-workers are a part. So you write down, to the best of your ability, what you think are the philosophy, goals and objectives for the organizational unit supervised by your own manager.

For your next step, you have several alternatives. The order in which you do them depends upon your own inclination, your knowledge of your own boss and subordinates, and how you size up the whole situation. Whatever the sequence, all of these steps will need to be carried out:

1. Discuss with your own personnel the philosophy and goals (as you understand them) of the entire organization unit of which you all are a part.
2. Develop with your own people a simple statement of the philosophy and goals of your own unit. (If such a statement already exists, review it with your employee group to determine what each one thinks it means to them in their own jobs.)
3. Develop with your own people a series of specific objectives for the months ahead. These should relate, insofar as possible, to your understanding of the objectives for the entire department or hospital.
4. Take to your boss, for discussion and approval, the list of written objectives you have developed with your people. Review what you have been doing. Say something like this: "We have based our own statements upon the philosophy, goals, and objectives of the hospital

(or institution or agency) and of the department (nursing service, maternal and child care or whatever) as we understand them. We used these statements as our guide for these."

Show and discuss what you have available for the philosophy, goals and objectives of the larger organizational unit. Obtain agreement, modified as necessary, that your statements of the foregoing are adequate as a starting point for what follows. Then say:

"Here are the statements we have developed for our own philosophy, goals and objectives. You will note that the philosophy and goals are the same as, or only slightly modified from, the larger goals and philosophy we have just discussed. Our objectives are specific to our own area of responsibility, and relate directly to the broader institutional and departmental objectives. We will appreciate your comments and suggestions."

The outcome of such an effort on your part depends upon a number of factors. One of the most important of these factors is the motive force at work in your relationship with your boss. Thus what happens as a result of your initiative in taking the foregoing steps may be surprisingly satisfying or predictably disappointing. Regardless of the outcome, however, you will have established a new base from which to build toward what you want to accomplish as manager of your unit.

THE BIG PICTURE

Figure 3:2 portrays how all employees on all shifts of every unit of every department in the entire organization are a vital part of implementing objectives that have their focus on the goals of the organization — its purpose and reason for existing. Your examination of this diagram will help in comprehending the significance of an MBO program in relation to your role in patient care and in making PONS work well in your agency. In this connection, the value of MBO and the other management techniques will become clearer as we examine the ways you can use these techniques.

Here is an example of a program performance plan that relates the individual employee and unit objectives to those of the larger organizational segments. The hospital goal is: Provide a complete range of emergency, short term, acute healthcare services at optimal cost for the community within our service area.

Figure 3:2
The MBO Schematic Organizational Plan

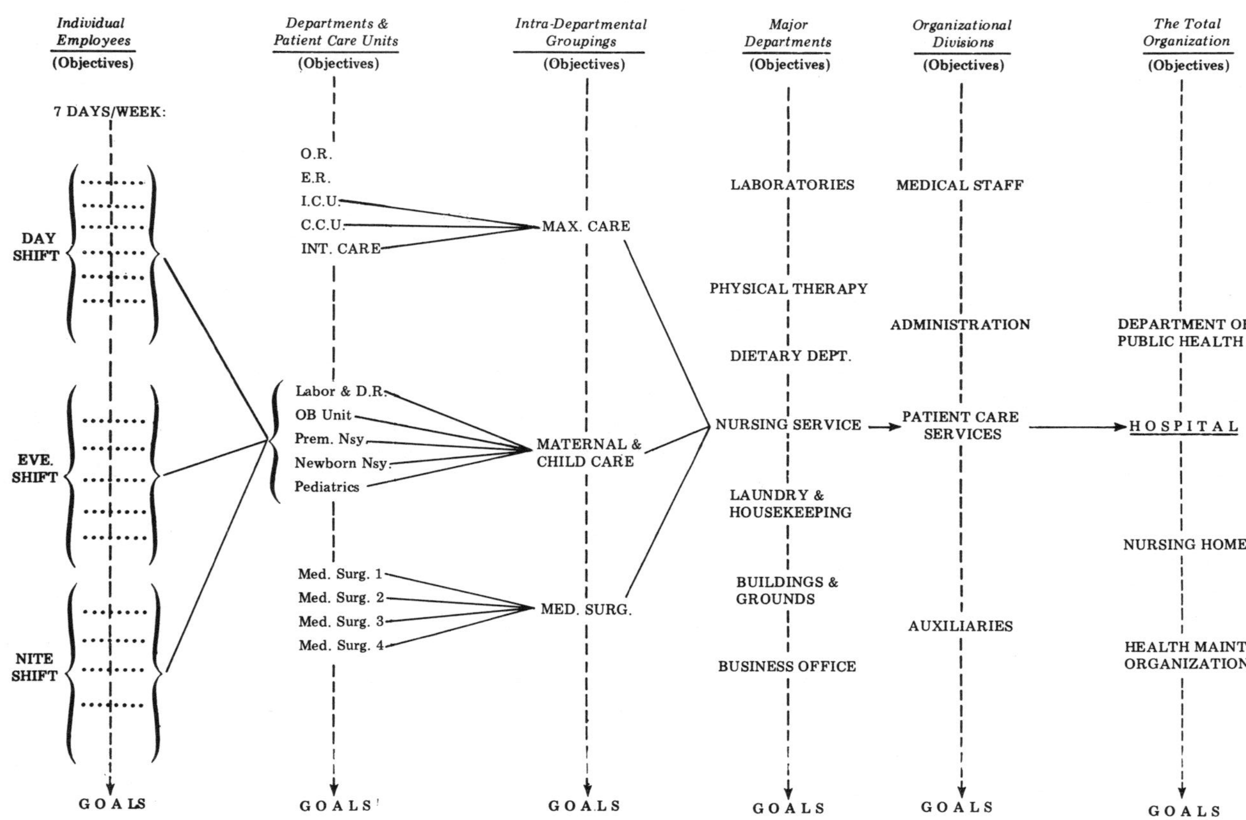

The picture presented is intended to explain MBO as a systematic, well organized process. It is a way of managing well—of planning, doing and controlling what has to be done. It will work as a systematic, well organized process when the people in an organization make it work that way for them.

UNIT OF ORGANIZATION	A SEQUENCE OF RELATED OBJECTIVES
Hospital (President or Administrator)	Expand the scope of maternal and child care services to provide a complete family centered program by June 30, 1977.
Medical Staff (President)	Present by September 1, 1975, the outline of an expanded patient care medical program in maternal and child care consonant with the goal of a complete family centered emphasis.
Dept. of Nursing Service (Dir. of Nursing Service)	Present by October 30, 1975 expanded nursing care program in maternal and child care consonant with the goal of a complete family centered emphasis.
Patient Care Services (Associate Administrator)	Integrate the planning of the OB/GYN/Peds section of the medical staff with the budget committee of the board of trustees, the facilities planning group and the director of nursing service; complete program performance plan by March 1, 1976.
Maternal & Child Care (Patient Care Coordinator)	Prepare specifications for the necessary equipment, facilities, supplies, and staffing to implement a complete nursing service program for family centered maternal and child care by December 31, 1976.
Obstetric Unit (Head Nurse) Labor & Del. (Head Nurse) Premy Nursery (Head Nurse) OB Nursery (Head Nurse) Pediatrics (Head Nurse)	Plan the details of initiating the expanded family-centered program as it affects the day to day operation of the unit; recruit and train additional personnel as required; reorient present staff to the concept and changed nursing requirements; schedule necessary implementation steps; complete plan by March 1, 1977.
Individuals (Nursing Staff) (Supervisors and/or Assoc. Directors of Nsg. Service; Eve., Nites, Weekends) (Employees of other affected hospital services)	Participate in planning as appropriate; assist in updating own performance description; contribute own suggestions; participate in reorientation program activities.

HELP WITH WRITING OBJECTIVES

An objective is a specific task-oriented statement of results to be achieved in order to accomplish a goal. Our objective in writing this section is to provide you with a model for writing objectives and with practice exercises so that when you have finished your reading and have done the exercises, by an established date you set for yourself, you will have acquired the skill to write meaningful objectives for your own work setting.

We have just seen one example of a program performance plan with a series of objectives, written by employees in a hierarchy of job levels, all pertaining to the same organizational goal. Here are three additional examples of objectives that fulfill the requirements for the inclusion of necessary components:

A. By an Inservice Education Director
Provide training and orientation for all newly hired groups of nursing school graduates so that they will be prepared to assume their job performance responsibilities by June 1.

B. By a Director of Nursing Service
Institute an effective problem-oriented system of charting on two selected patient care units by October 6, 1975, at a cost not to exceed the present unit cost per patient day for nursing service on these units.

C. By a Head Nurse
Adjust the staffing pattern and practices on my unit by January 1, 1976, so that the nursing hours per patient day, regardless of the patient census, do not vary more than plus or minus 5% from the established standard developed for my unit; and maintaining my flexibility to change the mix of nursing personnel classification if significant changes occur in the level of care required by a changing patient mix.

We find that in spite of so much emphasis on MBO during recent years, very few nurses have received instruction in how to write an objective. The following guidance will be of assistance. A meaningful written objective meets several important criteria. The written statements should include the following components: (1) What will be done? (2) How much will be done how well? (3) When will it be done? (4) Who will do what, where? (If pertinent) and (5) What will it cost? (If pertinent).

A useful exercise is to examine the first paragraph at the beginning of this section. Identify how our statement of objective for this section includes the foregoing components. Note any ways you would improve the statement so that it more clearly presents the components. This is a step toward helping you to remember the components. Next review the three examples of objectives by the inservice director, director of nursing service and head nurse. For each example identify the components by marking them with key words such as "what," "how much," "how well" over the appropriate portion of each objective. Compare your results with those of someone else. Now review again each of the components. Additional explanation of each one follows.

What will be done? The "what" portion of the objective begins with an active verb—provide, institute, adjust. The form of the statement is a simple declarative sentence: "Somebody does something." In the three examples, the "somebody" is understood; it is the "I" of the person in the job title. The "something" is the predicate. In example A, it is "training and orientation." In B, it is "an effective problem-oriented system of charting." In C, it is "the staffing pattern and practices."

How much will be done? This is the quantitative and qualitative component. This is frequently significant since it provides a measure of the degree of completeness of the finished objective.

In A: *All* new groups; will be *prepared*
In B: On *two* units; *no* increase in cost
In C: On *my* unit; *within plus or minus* 5% of standard; *flexibility* in mix of personnel categories.

When will it be done? This is the target date for completion. It is an essential item in every objective; it provides the basis for integrating a series of objectives (see examples of program performance plans). The target dates are necessary also for cash-flow planning in connection with budgets.

In A: June 1 (of each year)
In B: October 6, 1975
In C: January 1, 1976

Who will do what, where? (Optional) When the who and where are pertinent, later confusion and misunderstandings can be avoided by including names and places. These will be helpful too in preparing the program performance plan which needs to include identification of who will do, or help with, each implementation step.

In A: "I" implied; "In-house" implied
In B: "I" implied; two selected units
In C: "I" implied; my unit

What will it cost? (Optional) Every objective carries a cost that can be calculated. A cost effectiveness study in relation to an objective (or series of objectives) is simply an estimate of the financial cost of acheiving the objective compared with the expected financial benefits (income, savings, lowered expense) stemming from the implemented objective. Reference to cost may be included in the written statement when pertinent or required.

In A: None cited
In B: Not to exceed present unit cost/patient day (in operating cost)
In C: No installation cost; better control of wage cost (plus or minus 5% of standard) implied.

In your own planning you undoubtedly have some goals you want to achieve. What project do you want to get done in your unit that will contribute directly to the quality of patient care, better working conditions, or better control of expenses? Write a realistic, meaningful statement for a single objective in one of these three categories. Use each of the first three basic components, and include numbers 4 and 5 if appropriate. Identify and mark the components you have included, just as you did earlier for the examples.

THE NURSE MANAGER'S ROLE IN MBO

Making MBO work is a part of every manager's responsibility in every department, at every organizational level. Nurse managers are no exception. From director of nursing to head nurse, the nurse managers need to take the lead in using and guiding MBO. Their roles are especially important in hospitals, nursing homes and public health agencies since so many projects and objectives initiated in nursing service necessarily involve the participation of other hospital or agency department heads if the objectives are to be met successfully. The expansion or contraction of patient care programs has impact throughout the entire organization and often throughout the community, because of their relation to hospital goals and the competing demands for resources — personnel, money, facilities, equipment.

The organizational climate and its influence upon the motivation of all personnel is as important to the implementation of MBO as to other management-initiated programs. And it is the managers themselves who, more than anyone else, influence the organizational climate, employee morale and motivation. Myers presents a concept of job enrichment that permits each employee the maximum possible degree of planning and control of his work.[7] This is highly relevant as a useful concept to aid managers in using MBO. It influences the managerial style of managers and how they use their leadership skills. Consider how the performance results of your people reflect the degree of success you achieve in the leadership behaviors listed in the goal-oriented column of Figure 3:3. Evaluate yourself for your level of ability in performing, regularly, each of the eight items using a scale with a plus for "very well;" a check mark for "OK, as well as I'd expect;" and a dash for "less satisfactorily than I'd like." Relate this self-evaluation to your own level of motivation for using MBO as part of your nurse-manager responsibilities and functions.

Figure 3:3
The Role Of The Manager

Authority-Oriented	Goal-Oriented
Set goals for subordinates, define standards and results expected.	Participate with people in problem solving and goal setting.
Give them information necessary to do their jobs.	Give them access to information which they want.
Train them to do the job.	Create situations for optimum learning.
Explain rules and apply discipline to ensure conformity; suppress conflict.	Explain rules and consequences of violations; mediate conflict.
Stimulate subordinates through persuasive leadership.	Allow people to set challenging goals.
Develop and install new methods.	Teach methods improvement techniques to job incumbents.
Develop and free them for promotion.	Enable them to pursue and move into growth opportunities.
Reward achievements and punish failures.	Recognize achievements and help them learn from failures.

From M. Scott Myers, <u>Every Employee A Manager</u> (New York: McGraw-Hill, 1970), p. 99.

DEVELOPING A PROGRAM PERFORMANCE PLAN

A program performance plan (PPP) is a long-range schedule of inter-related steps required to effect a desired result, objective or goal. It is a planning tool. "Planning" is thinking ahead, determining what shall be done; the management function of establishing goals, setting objectives, defining problems and opportunities, and developing strategy and tactics for achieving objectives.

A graphic portrayal of a PPP is shown in Figure 3:4. The first example is one we prepared for an operations appraisal project within a large county Board of Health. You may wish to construct your own plan using the sequence of objectives found on page 82. There are many advantages to using a graphic chart showing weeks and months of the year. The benefits of this format are that it:

1. Permits seeing at a glance the timetable for beginning and completing each step.
2. Shows the interrelationships of the steps (and objectives) with other scheduled events (holidays, budget submission, vacations, etc.).
3. Provides (in column at right margin) for including names of who will do or help with each step.
4. Emphasizes the variety of demands upon manager's time, and helps to avoid overly optimistic target dates for completion.
5. Communicates the schedule to others in a form easy to understand.
6. Is highly flexible and adaptable to inclusion of other dates, color coding, revisions, progress notes and symbols.

Here are some tips to remember in connection with establishing the target dates for each step. A person inexperienced in setting up such a schedule is inclined to begin from today's date with the first step and plan forward with each succeeding step. A better plan is to use a worksheet, and start by listing the last step you visualize prior to the target date for completing the objective. Then, working backwards to the present time of year, list each preceding step with its beginning and ending date based upon your best estimate of the work involved. When this is done realistically, you may be surprised to discover that already, as of the present date, you are overdue for beginning the first step. Psychologically, this working backwards from the last step to the first seems to help avoid the temptation, having established the target

Figure 3:4
Sample Operations Appraisal
Program Performance Plan

ACTIVITIES	1973								
	JUNE				JULY				
	11 12 13 14 15	18 19 20 21 22	25 26 27 28 29	2 3 (4) 5 6	9 10 11 12 13	16 17 18 19 20	23 24 25 26 27		
Phase I	◄——————————— P H A S E I ———————————►								
1. Orientation Meetings with Dept. Heads									
2. Departmental Interviews	Individuals and Groups								
3. On-the-Job Observations		Selective review of job activities							
4. Ratio-Delay Analysis (selected jobs)			Continuing observation						
5. Program Analyses	Identification of goals, standards, and preliminary evaluation								
6. Functional Analysis				Management style; systems, controls					
7. Data Analysis	On-going accumulation and evaluation of selective data								
8. Phase I Progress Report						Report Prep. & Presentation			
Phase II									
9. Implementation, from Phase I Rec.									
10. Self-Development Program									
11. Opinion Surveys (optional)									
12. Annual Business Plan; Final Report									

Figure 3:4 (Cont.)

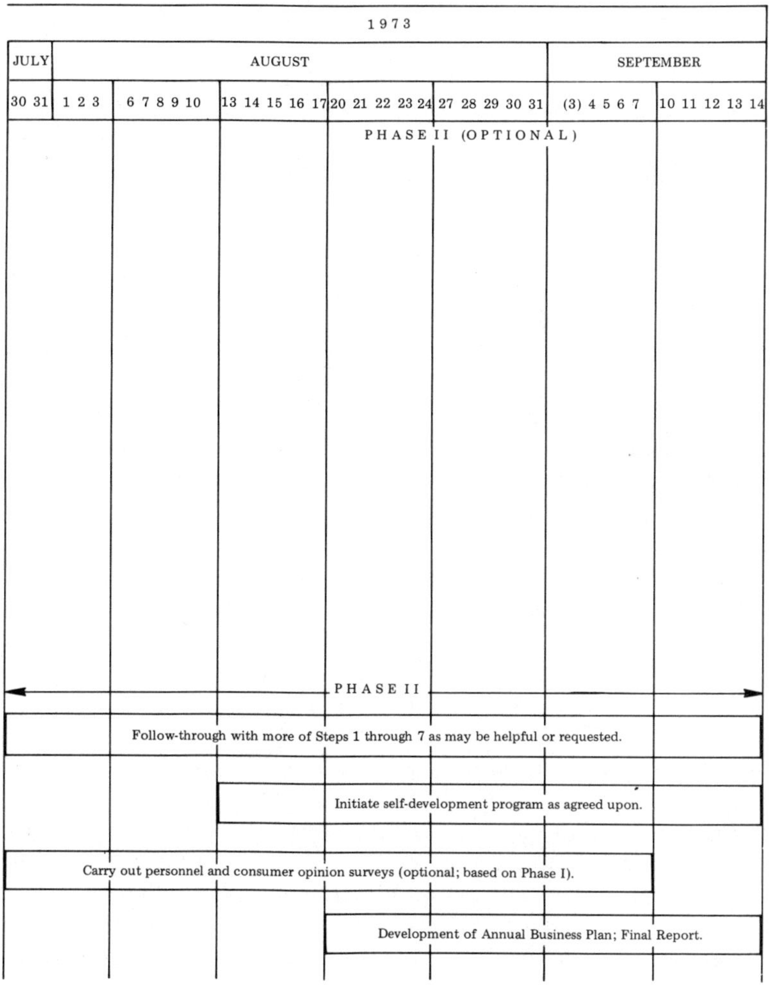

	1973							
JULY	AUGUST					SEPTEMBER		
30 31	1 2 3	6 7 8 9 10	13 14 15 16 17	20 21 22 23 24	27 28 29 30 31	(3) 4 5 6 7	10 11 12 13 14

PHASE II (OPTIONAL)

PHASE II

Follow-through with more of Steps 1 through 7 as may be helpful or requested.

Initiate self-development program as agreed upon.

Carry out personnel and consumer opinion surveys (optional; based on Phase I).

Development of Annual Business Plan; Final Report.

date for completion, of unrealistically compressing the time schedule for each step. Too often the end target date is established prior to thinking through the details of all the work involved in carrying out the objective. When the final schedule is transferred to the PPP form, the steps will be listed in calendar sequence from top to bottom for ease of use and comprehension.

Another approach is to write on separate cards all of the steps you can visualize as they occur to you, in no particular order. Then arrange the cards in the sequence in which you think the steps should be taken. Finally, assign the projected starting and ending dates for each step.

MBO AND NMBO

NMBO is Nursing Management by Objectives. It is MBO as applied by nurse *managers* as part of their management responsibilities for personnel, facilities, patient care, budgetary planning and control within their own segments of the nursing department. The term NMBO is used herein to distinguish it from NBO—Nursing by Objectives—which is the application of MBO to the management of direct patient care by individual RNs and team leaders, the *nurse* managers.

To clarify the emphasis of NMBO, a review of the scope of nurse manager responsibilities will be helpful. These are presented in Part 1 where the Workworld of the Nurse Manager shows the three major areas of responsibility as comprising patient care management, operational management and human resources management. These are not three distinct, separate areas of responsibility. They necessarily overlap, merge and harmonize in the interests of nursing, patient care and organizational goals.

Management by objectives is simply one of several techniques used by nurses at all organizational levels to assist in bringing about this harmony of effort toward achieving mutual goals. The scope of the nurse manager's application of NMBO, therefore, is greater and for a wider variety of purposes than the applications to be made by a staff nurse. All nurses, however, are expected to use the elements of the management process as they pertain to each nurse's performance responsibilities (see Appendices A and G).

ROPEP AND MBO

One of the other management techniques that works hand-in-hand with NMBO is a results-oriented performance evaluation program (ROPEP).

"Plan for MBO" (Figure 3:2) shows the sequence of steps in translating the hospital (or organization-wide) goals and objectives into performance responsibilities and objectives for individual employees. The diagram is expanded in Figure 3:5 to show how the techniques of MBO and ROPEP combine to produce the desired performance results and goal achievement. The ROPEP cycle involves: first, Identifying for Whom Major Performance Responsibilities are Performed; second, Writing the Segments of Performance Responsibilities; and third, Developing the Performance Standards for each Segment. The MBO cycle involves: first, Setting Mutual Goals and Objectives; then, Performing the Necessary Activities to Achieve the Objectives; and finally, Reviewing Progress and Evaluating Achievements. Note the significance of the continuation of the sequence. This emphasizes the importance of developing the individual performance descriptions before setting mutual goals and performance descriptions with those individuals who will participate. Objectives are carried out by people as part of their regular performance responsibilities. Thus the measure of achievement in meeting objectives is not an evaluation exercise separate from regular performance evaluation. Successful carrying out of individual performance responsibilities leads to successful achievement of objectives—and of the goals to which such objectives are related.

The foregoing is true even in those cases when out-of-the-ordinary projects and special assignments are necessary. Some projects and assignments may be agreed upon for the purpose of challenging or expanding the capabilities of the person involved. It may be a part of that person's growth and development program in connection with both individual and organizational goals. Even when such assignments are part of a person's preparation for assuming a position of greater responsibility, the activities related to such projects are necessarily a part of a person's current performance responsibilities.

The shaded area marked "Revisions" in Figure 3:5 is that portion of the ROPEP/MBO cycles where they overlap. It is that portion of the introductory/implementation/follow-through phases of performance evaluation and MBO which provides for making necessary revisions in the tools and procedures. Performance requirements change; statements of satisfactory performance have to be updated; objectives have to be modified, eliminated, expanded or replaced. Such revisions are essential and must be made as soon as their need is identified,

Figure 3:5
ROPEP & MBO: A Functional Diagram

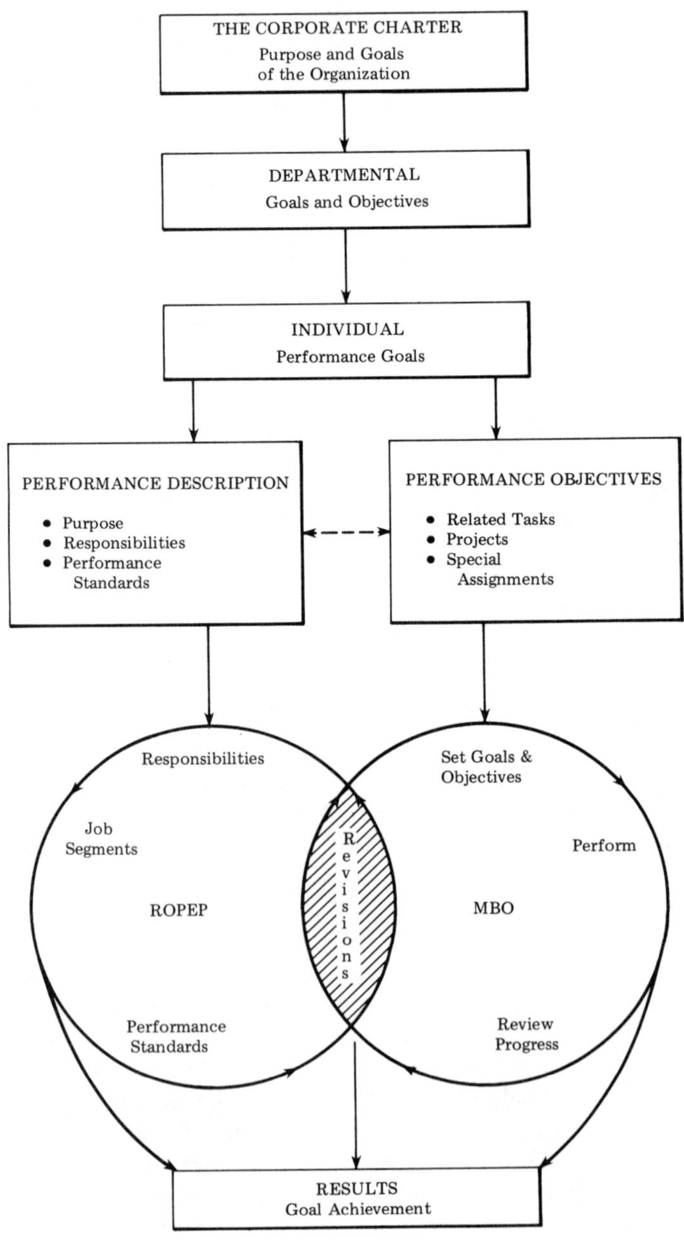

rather than being accumulated for an annual or semiannual updating process. ROPEP and MBO provide nurse managers with important tools and techniques for daily use in their managing process. Most tools require regular maintenance, whether they are clinical tools (stethoscopes, monitors, blood pumps) or management tools (performance description, written objective, program performance plan). If they do not receive regular care and maintenance they do not work well and impair the nurse manager's performance.

In short, the lower portion of the diagram shows both ROPEP and MBO as management techniques being used by nurse managers in carrying out their management functions of planning, doing and controlling. Thus a performance evaluation discussion by a nurse manager and a staff worker involves not only a review of the performance results of the employee in carrying out the regular performance responsibilities, but also a review of progress and results on previously agreed-upon objectives.

Results are produced by people. Some results are achieved through efforts and activities that are part of a person's regular day-to-day performance responsibilities in the job. Other results are attained primarily through an extra quota of effort and the effective performance of special projects and task assignments.[8] ROPEP and MBO, together, provide the techniques, stimulus and evaluative methods for securing optimum results through both types of individual effort.

The outcomes of this process hoped for are results that contribute to achievement of the purposes of the individual employee, the department and the organization. In hospitals and other healthcare agencies, the expected beneficiaries are the consumers themselves.

The Objectives Worksheet

Another tool for use with both MBO and ROPEP is the Objectives Worksheet. (Figure 3:6). This form supplements the program performance plan and the performance description. It can be used to plan and evaluate the performance of special tasks and assignments that are part of carrying out a specific objective. The objectives worksheet can be used also to plan and evaluate objectives that are generated as a follow through to a discussion of job-connected performance results that are less than satisfactory.

An examination of the Objectives Worksheet shows that it is a larger and different version of the MBO cyclical diagram, expanded to serve as an $8\frac{1}{2}$" x 11" worksheet. One of these worksheets prepared for each objective serves as a planning and evaluative tool in connec-

Figure 3:6

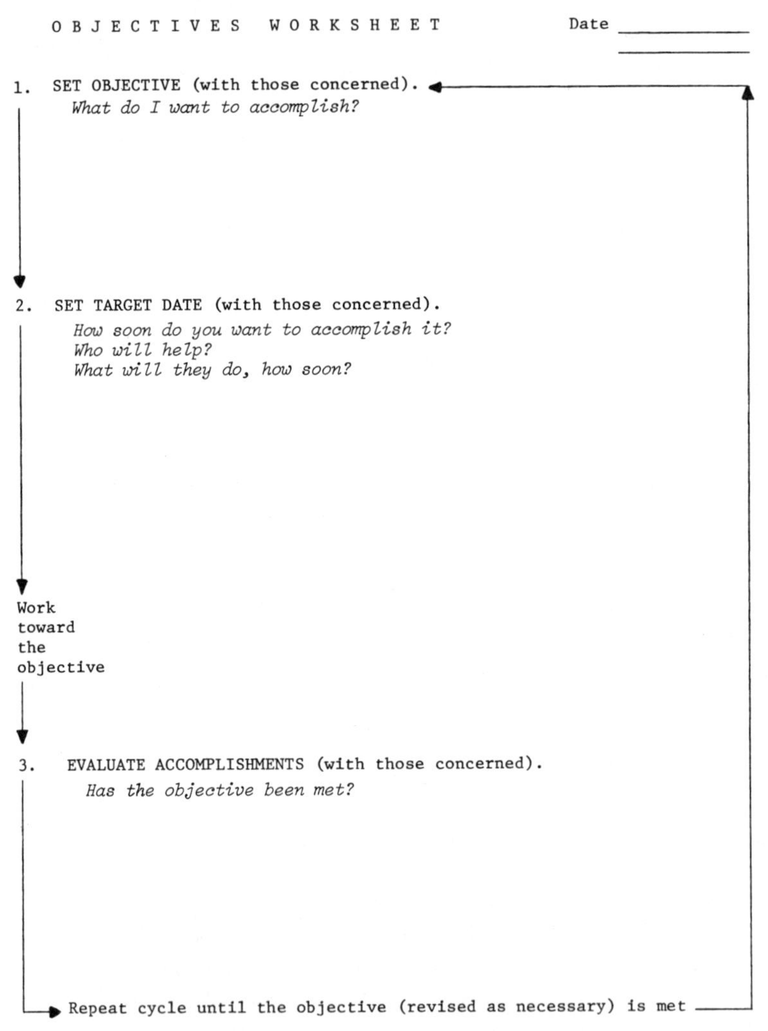

tion with discussions between a person and his boss. Each worksheet remains active for the life of the objective to which it pertains. It is revised as required or when target dates have to be extended. When an objective is terminated for whatever reason (successful completion, cancelled due to budgetary curtailment, phased out or merged with another project), the related worksheet, properly annotated, becomes a historical record for follow through purposes.

NMBO And Other Management Techniques

Nurse managers who develop familiarity and skill with NMBO quickly learn its value as a kind of master coordinating tool for other aspects and techniques of nurse management. These include patient care program development, nursing audit, problem-oriented nursing system, wide-track careers planning, handling complaints and grievances, motivational management, personnel development and annual budgetary planning and control.

Annual budgetary planning (ABP) is used here as an example which, like ROPEP and MBO, reflects the cyclical three steps of plan, do and control. From some points of view,budgetary planning represents the ultimate application of MBO. This is because the budgetary planning process, when properly carried out, necessarily:

— builds upon the short and long range program plans that
— generate the objectives that
— create demands for resource allocation that
— must be translated into dollars in a proposed budget.

Later, the approved budget (i.e., a schedule for spending) becomes an MBO document that:

— permits securing the resources (personnel, equipment, supplies, facilities, education and training) to
— carry out objectives that
— implement programs (for patients, personnel, the community) that
— fulfill the organizational goals.

A later chapter provides a detailed explanation of ABP as a nurse-manager technique.

Securing Involvement

By definition, MBO is a technique that includes the preparation of mutually established objectives. ROPEP, for example, involves preparing agreed-upon standards of performance. Other management techniques also require the participation and involvement of personnel with their own managers in the development of standards and objectives, and in evaluating performance results.

The word "involve" by definition means to include, draw in, embroil, engross. The word "participate" by definition means to take part, join, share. For human beings generally, the foregoing types of action are natural tendencies (until learned behavior seems to indicate otherwise). Yet many nurse managers appear to be uneasy with, or unskilled in, the process of securing meaningful involvement. The reasons often include the fact that they really don't know how to do it; they haven't learned the skills; they have had no model to follow (no boss of their own who has ever been a skilled facilitator); or they see no reason for trying.

A major reason for securing involvement in the processes we have described is that better performance results can be obtained by doing so. At least this has been the experience of many nurse managers. They often discover also that they enjoy their managing more. In addition, employees at every level can meet some of their human needs and achieve greater job satisfaction through meaningful participation and involvement.

You can secure more involvement and participation by your people through use of the following suggestions:

1. Act as though you want your people involved.

Never be too busy to listen (even though it takes time) or your people will think you really don't want to hear them or involve them.

2. Ask for help. (Invite participation).

There once was a nurse manager who, whenever she was asked by an LPN what to do about a patient problem, would tell the LPN what to do. One day when the LPN asked about how to handle another problem, the nurse manager asked, "What do you think?"

"Huh?" responded the LPN, in a mild state of shock. "I asked you to tell me how you think you can solve it," said the nurse manager.

"That's what I thought you said,'" answered the LPN, "But I didn't think you really meant it." Then the LPN proceeded to give her own idea, was encouraged to try it, and it worked.

3. Use "Tips for Leading Discussions."

These tips may help you, as they have others, to get good results in leading group discussions. They work well also in face-to-face discussions with another person as in interviews, performance evaluation and problem solving (These "tips" can be found in *HELP with Management by Objectives*, number 4, by Joan and Warren Ganong.)

What is management? It is the process of getting meaningful results through and with other people. NMBO helps to do it better. Securing successful involvement is a key to NMBO.

The NBO Concept

Managing patient care is different from managing personnel who are members of a patient care unit. The differences are both in kind and degree of activity. Managing unit personnel involves assigning care for the entire group of patients. This is the basic concept, even though it may be modified depending upon the setting and the nurse manager. Managing patient care involves the concept of one nurse and one patient working together to carry out the medical care plan and the nursing care plan for that patient. While this concept can rarely be implemented without modification, application efforts to carry out the concept are being made by nurses with such titles as nurse practitioner, primary nurse and clinical specialist.

Nursing by Objectives is a results-oriented technique using mutually-established patient care objectives, an implementation schedule, and evaluation of results and patient progress. It applies the management-by-objectives approach at the unit level with the focus on the one nurse/one patient relationship. The emphasis is not the performance of tasks for patients. It is upon helping the patient achieve his goals. This means establishing a helping relationship between nurse and patient, a relationship in which the patient is recognized as being in charge of himself (insofar as he is able) and the nurse is a facilitative manager of goal achievement in accordance with the medical care plan.

The following list summarizes the purpose of NBO and the variety of factors that influence how well the patient and the nurse can work together to achieve their mutual objectives. Very likely you can add additional factors which will influence the patient/nurse interaction and how well the goals are met.

INFLUENCING FACTORS

Patient	*Nurse*
Own human needs	Own human needs
Specific health problems	Medical plan of care

INFLUENCING FACTORS (Cont.)

Patient	*Nurse*
Medical care plan	Nursing care plan
Family involvement	Discharge planning
Degree of dependency	Teaching process
Learning process	Organizational environment
Others	Others

By using mutual understanding, trust, cooperation, and skill the goals of both the nurse and patient can be achieved.

The foregoing introduction to nursing by objectives is intended to help develop an awareness of the shift in emphasis in using NBO as contrasted with NMBO. Both are management techniques to assist in achieving patient care goals. But NBO is more specifically and directly related to the nursing process for each individual person. NBO, therefore, becomes an integral part of assessing, planning, implementing and evaluating each person's needs and plan of care. Think of it as a series of concentric circles cyclic in nature with NBO at the center as the specific management technique; the nursing process as the outer circle; and the middle circle as the integrating model of the management process.

Some of the similarities and distinctions between NMBO and NBO are summarized below. An understanding of this comparison summary will assist all nursing unit personnel to participate easily and effectively in the use of management by objectives.

Table 3:2
Comparison Summary

Feature	NMBO	NBO
Aim	Goal Achievement	Goal Achievement
Focus	Personnel Management	Patient Care Management
Method	MBO Technique	MBO Technique
Objectives	Oriented to nursing management objectives	Oriented to direct patient care objectives
Motivation	Self (Nursing Personnel)	Self (Patient)
Involvement	Nurse Managers/Personnel	Nursing Personnel/ Patient/Family
Process	Problem Solving/Unit Management	Problem Solving/ Nursing Process

An Example of Interrelated Goals

Dorothea E. Orem has written, "The nurse's special interest is the continuing therapeutic care which the patient requires....The nursing focus takes into account both the medical point of view and the patient's point of view."[9]

The implementation of NBO takes into account the goals and objectives of the patient's doctor, together with three other aspects of nursing goals and objectives. These three aspects are (1) Your own, as the patient's nurse; (2) The patient's, as a person; (3) The family's, as healthcare consumers.

Here is an example of three short-range goals for a married female patient, age 40, who has successfully undergone the surgical intervention and initial recovery phases of an abdominal hysterectomy. The patient's goal is to move about without pain. The husband's goal is to reassure his wife that she is still loved and needed; and the nurse's goal is to prevent circulatory complications.

Note that these are all goals each person sets for himself—the patient, as self; the husband, as self; and the nurse, as self. All are meaningful and need attention. The nurse needs to be aware of all three goals with an understanding that, while each person can set objectives to meet parts of each of the goals, no one person can meet all of the goals. It will require the patient, husband, doctor and nurse— working together—to satisfy all these goals. For patient-care objectives to be practical at the direct care level, it is necessary to determine selectively which of the components of an objective are appropriate and useful in a given situation. Let's follow through with the three separate goals and see what objectives might assist the three parties involved to achieve those goals.

The patient's goal is to move about without pain. One of the patient's objectives might be to learn to support the area of incision with her hands during the first 48-hour postoperative period. A second patient objective is to request a pain medication 20 minutes before attempting to get out of bed (for three postoperative days).

The husband's objectives can be (1) to demonstrate on each visit, through words and attitude, his continuing love, devotion and need for his wife, and (2) to remind and assist her in her pain-control practices. And the nurse, to meet the goal of preventing circulatory complications has an objective to schedule and assign staff to help the patient increase the number of occasions for exercise at regular intervals on each successive postoperative day.

Note that the husband's objectives, if carefully set and carried out, help to meet his needs as well as his wife's needs and goals. Similarly the nurse, in setting and carrying out his/her objectives, will help achieve his/her goal while facilitating both husband and wife in meeting their objectives—and hence in meeting their goals. But this kind of mutually satisfying outcome is not likely to be achieved if the several persons involved set their goals and objectives independently of one another.

As we learn more and more to include the patient and family in the patient's care we need to practice the setting of mutual goals. Setting goals with instead of for people may take place between the doctor and nurse, the doctor and patient, the nurse and the patient, the patient and family, and any combination of the above individuals as the patient's needs indicate. This mutual goal setting must be documented. Appropriate places can be provided in the patient's medical record for this documentation. The goals that involve the nursing staff with patient and family may be noted on the nursing care plan as in the example (Exhibit 3:1). In this example the goals are based upon the needs and problems of the patient. Specific approaches are then identified on the nursing care plan to meet each need or problem.

Exhibit 3:1
Nursing Care Plan

GOAL: Prepare patient to return home. Create and maintain therapeutic environment. Maintain good hygiene and physical comfort

DATE	PROBLEMS AND NEEDS	APPROACH
1	Requires medication for pain q 2-3 hrs	Give medication as ordered. Turn, cough and deep breathe.
2	Abd. incision draining slightly	Observe and report condition of wound.
3	Indwelling cath.	Measure and record urinary drainage
4	Intake and output	Keep accurate intake and output
5	Requires assistance in getting O.O.B.	Assist out of bed.
6	Observe for abdominal distention	Patient may need rectal tube or enema as ordered.
7	Poor sleeping habits at home	Observe and report sleep pattern. Offer back care and refreshments when awake.
8	Crying at times	Facilitate awareness of self as an individual with varying physical, emotional and developmental needs.

Age	Birth Date	S(M)DW	Religion	Profession	Adm	Date
44	05-04-30		pro	NIP		

Room	NAME		DIAGNOSIS	DOCTOR
224			Abd. Hysterectomy	

NBO and PONS

When a person enters today's healthcare system for care, that person assumes the role of patient. Similarly, when people enter the workforce in any healthcare organization, they assume the role designated by their titles. But each of us has many roles in our life and work. And whatever role each of us may assume, we bring ourselves into the situation as persons. Goals and objectives are set by persons. Systems are designed by persons. But a technique or system is only as effective as the person who uses it. This is as true for NBO as it is for any other technique or process. We believe that nurses can make a conscious decision to identify meaningful goals and objectives mutually with doctors, patients and families—and with other healthcare personnel. Regardless of the pressures brought to bear on nurses by the organization in which they work, only the nurses themselves can ultimately decide to set mutual goals and objectives, professionally, or not to do so.

If you are like many nurses you can recall one or more occasions when you have made a statement such as the following: "Oh, I can't do that. I can't learn to practice MBO. I just can't be a manager." The next time you say, or are tempted to say, "I can't" change it to "I won't do that; I won't learn to, etc." Nearly always the "I won't'" is a more accurate statement than the "I can't." As a prepared nurse you can do almost anything you really want to do—if you are willing to pay the price in time, effort and the learning of newer knowledge and skills. If you can visualize how the consequences of what you decide you can do are better care for your patients, and greater work satisfaction for yourself, you are likely to want to pay the price in return for the benefits. In economic and budgetary terminology, the translation of such a comparison into quantitative measures is known as the price/benefit ratio. As Katherine B. Nuckolls has said, "Ultimately, the person who really determines what the nurse can do is the nurse herself. Her perception of her role and her expectations of herself will be the most important determinants of her behavior."[10]

NBO and PONS are two techniques or systems that complement one another. Table 3:3 is a summary comparison of the basic components of both, presented in the context of the management functions of plan, do and control.

Table 3:3

Comparison of NBO and PONS

NBO	PLAN	PONS
Set a goal	P L A N	Principles of practice
Set objectives		The nursing process
Work toward the objectives and goals	D O	Problem/oriented nursing record
Evaluate level of achievement of goals and objectives	C O N T R O L	Nursing audit Nursing inservice and continuing education

Human Mode and Technical Mode in MBO

Clearly the emphasis of MBO as presented herein is upon the human elements as much as upon the technical aspects of the subject. This is necessarily so. MBO is not a new program or system to be superimposed upon an existing organizational way of getting results. MBO provides, however, a possible new outlook, a different way of seeking the accomplishment of the major purposes of the agency and its subdivisions. It also points the way to the need for sharpening the skills of managers who have the responsibility for getting results — through the use of MBO and such additional techniques as the managers use in carrying out their functions.

Nurses are in the fortunate position of being able to accommodate the principles and practices of MBO quite readily. MBO fits a familiar pattern of the nurses' educational preparation. It is consistent with the nursing process. It is easily adapted to nurse manager responsibilities via NMBO and to patient care management responsibilities via NBO. The revelation for some nurses that "Why, this is very much like what I have been doing all along!" may come as a surprise. Such a reaction can be helpful or hurtful; helpful, if it leads to more skillful use of MBO to strengthen present practices in personnel and patient care management, but hurtful if it leads to thinking MBO has nothing to offer nurses, the nursing department or patients. MBO has much to offer because it can become the means toward greater agency-wide cooperation and effectiveness.

Agency-Wide Use of MBO

In many healthcare organizations, the method of introducing MBO and other management techniques has been based upon a business or industrial model. Examples used in MBO orientation and training sessions have in many health agency applications been selected from business or nonpatient-care situations.

We have reversed the customary approach. We have presented MBO as a technique for nurse managers. An obvious reason for this is to increase the likelihood of understanding, acceptance and use by nurses of this valuable method for managing. Another vital reason is the fact that the nursing department in the typical hospital spends upwards of forty per cent (40%) of the institution's operating expenses each year. In addition, the day-to-day patient care activities of the nursing department reach out to involve all other departments of the organization. Finally, nursing departments are often led by excellent managers; and it is the best managers who most often can see the value of an improved technique or method, who will adopt it and use it in the interest of high-quality, optimum-cost patient care.

Marvin Weisbord has put some of these considerations into sharp focus. He writes:

> ...consider a connection between deteriorating doctor-nurse relationships and rising hospital costs. There are in the main three things hospital patients need: Clinical care, personal attention, and help in getting a complex system to focus on their own case. Doctors provide the first service. Increasingly, aides do the "hands-on" care, clerks the paperwork, allied technicians the clinical tests, and ombudsmen the patient advocacy. Nurses, who might provide a link between clinical and administrative tasks are being squeezed out. RN's often don't want the narrow jobs, for they are trained to greater responsibility.
>
> They cannot use their knowledge well in the present setup, despite the fact they spend more time with patients, and often understand better than anyone the complex relationship among physical, emotional, social and administrative problems. With clinical and administrative training, they might make excellent hospital integrators—much better, in fact, than doctors or administrators. Instead, they are opting for the Identity game—seeking to become nurse practitioners—because nobody, themselves included, can visualize a more appropriate use for their training.[11]

It should be clear that we believe that nurse managers sometimes are, and certainly can become, "excellent hospital integrators." This is most likely to happen only when all management members of the healthcare team understand each other's roles and cooperate with those persons — nurse managers or others — who are willing and able to assume the hospital integrator responsibility.

Experience has demonstrated that all hospital department heads are usually willing and able to benefit from management development efforts that focus on management functions, techniques and skills. Department heads learn to conceptualize and understand their managerial roles better, to enjoy their work more, and to contribute more effectively to the goals of the hospital. MBO is one such technique that deserves agency-wide understanding, strong implementation leadership from the chief executive, and consistent follow-through as part of day-to-day management. MBO serves as as a method for integrating personal and departmental objectives. MBO facilitates interdisciplinary efforts to achieve the broad goals of individuals and the healthcare agency. MBO works best when it is used in this manner, rather than being carried out as a separate program apart from the day-to-day use of the management process. Subsequent chapters present additional management techniques — performance evaluation, nursing audit, budgetary planning — from the same point of view. They work best when used within the same framework of concepts and philosophy as MBO. Altogether, these techniques help nurse managers to carry out their management functions.

NOTES

1. Peter M. Drucker, *Management: Tasks, Responsibilities, Practices* (New York:McGraw-Hill, Inc., 1974), pp. 441-442. Excerpt reprinted with permission.

2. Marie DiVincenti, *Administering Nursing Service* (Boston: Little, Brown, and Co., 1972), p.75.

3. Douglas McGregor, *The Human Side of Enterprise* (New York: McGraw Hill, Inc., 1960).

4. E. Wight Bakke, "Teamwork in Industry," *The Scientific Monthly*, 66 (March 1948), pp. 213-220.

5. Douglas McGregor, *The Professional Manager* (New York: McGraw-Hill, Inc., 1967). © 1967 by McGraw-Hill, Inc. Used with permission of McGraw-Hill Book Company.

6. A.W. Combs, D.L. Avila and W.W. Purkey, *Helping Relationships: Basic Concepts for the Helping Professions* (Boston: Allyn and Bacon, 1971), p.165.

7. M. Scott Myers, *Every Employee a Manager* (New York: McGraw-Hill, Inc., 1970), pp. 69-70.

8. For a brief explanation of the project management concept, see Johnson, G.V. and Tingey, S., "Matrix Organization: Blueprint of Nursing Care Organization for the 80s,"*Hospital & Health Services Administration,* Winter, 1976, pp.27-39.

9. Dorothea E. Orem, *Nursing: Concepts of Practice* (New York: McGraw-Hill,Inc., 1971), p.49.

10. Katherine B. Nuckolls, "Who Decides What the Nurse Can Do?" *Nursing Outlook,* 22 (October 1974), p.630.

11. Marvin R. Weisbord, "Why Organization Development Hasn't Worked (So Far) in Medical Centers," *Health Care Management Review,* 1 (Spring 1976), p. 26. Excerpt reprinted with permission of Aspen Systems Corporation.

SUGGESTED READINGS

Books

Bakke, E. Wight. *The Bonds of Organization: An Appraisal of Corporate Human Relations* (Hamden, Conn.: Archon Books, 1966).

Combs, A.W.; Avila, D.L.; and Purkey, W.W. *Helping Relationships: Basic Concepts for the Helping Profession* (Boston: Allyn & Bacon, 1971).

Cornuelle, Richard. *De-Managing America—The Final Revolution* (New York: Random House, 1975).

DiVincenti, Marie. *Administering Nursing Services* (Boston: Little, Brown, and Co. 1972).

Drucker, Peter F. *Management: Tasks, Responsibilities, Practices* (New York, 1974).

Ganong, Joan and Warren. *HELP with Management by Objectives* (Chapel Hill, N.C.: W.L. Ganong, Co. 1975).

Morrisey, George. *Management by Objectives and Results* (Reading, Mass.: Addison Wesley Publishing Co., 1970).

Myers, M. Scott, *Every Employee a Manager: More Meaningful Work through Job Enrichment* (New York: McGraw-Hill, Inc., 1970).

Odiorne, George. *Management by Objectives* (New York: Pitman Publishing Co., 1965).

Odiorne, George. *Management Decision by Objectives* (Englewood Cliffs, N.J.: Prentice-Hall, 1969).

Article

Sherwin, Douglas S., "Management *of* Objectives," *Harvard Business Review,* 54 (May-June 1976).

Chapter 4
A Results-Oriented Performance Evaluation Program

"HOW AM I DOING?"

All members of a nursing staff need to know how they are doing. You and others have a right to receive answers to the often-voiced questions, "Where do I stand?" and "Is my work OK?" You may get answers from the people you are working for—the patients, the doctors, your own nurse supervisor, someone in administration, or other personnel. When any of these people tell you, "You've done a good job!", you feel great. You like praise because it satisfies your basic need for a true sense of self-worth, self-respect, status, ego satisfaction.

You hurt if you are deprived of this kind of need satisfaction. You probably feel this hurt just as much as when you are deprived of other basic biological requirements for remaining healthy—such as the need for air, water and food. If you are told, "That was a poor job," or "You really made a bad mistake," or "Why can't you do it right?", you are likely to feel badly. You hurt. You hurt because one of your basic human needs has been assaulted. Other employees, given similar messages, respond in much the same way as you. This is a simple fact whether or not the persons involved comprehend the significance of Maslow's hierarchy of human needs and their influence upon motivation as described in Appendix I. But every nurse manager in today's healthcare agencies should understand and be able to use the human need theory of motivation.

Consider the strength of your own emotional reactions when your nurse manager tells you positive or negative things about yourself or your work. Then it really is "for counts." You react to negative criticism with identifiable feelings even when you know that such criticism is justified. You, like other people, have a fairly accurate idea of how well you are doing your job. You feel it inside yourself when you have done a good day's work. And you usually know it, without anyone telling you, when you have blundered. But what is most disheartening is when the boss gives you an evaluation which disagrees with your own honest evaluation of yourself. And other people, under similar circumstance, feel very much as you do.

This is a problem. It is a problem in many hospitals because of the awkward situation in which the department heads and nurse managers find themselves. They know they are required or expected to evaluate the employees they supervise. But they often are frustrated, uncomfortable, even hostile to the whole routine because they know or feel that:

- The existing evaluation procedure is inadequate for its purpose.
- The techniques for evaluation are unsatisfactory for measuring results.
- They are not sufficiently familiar with the performance of the person being evaluated.
- They lack training in the necessary interviewing and counseling skills.
- They have insufficient time to do evaluations.
- Their guilt feelings tend to make them angry with the people they must evaluate.

In such circumstances it is no wonder that nurse managers often resent the time and effort devoted to personnel evaluations, and that the intended purpose of the evaluation process is served so poorly. In St. Joseph Hospital, St. Paul, we asked a group of twenty head nurses, who had already expressed their dissatisfaction with the existing employee appraisal form, to respond to these questions: "How would you design a performance evaluation plan? What characteristics should it have? What conditions should such a plan satisfy?" These head nurses, working in nondirected, simultaneous knee-group discussions, developed a significant number of recommendations and criteria for such a performance evaluation plan in less than one-half hour. They felt that such a plan should provide for self-evaluation, not just an evaluation by one's own nurse manager; evaluations should be scheduled more often than once per year; the evaluation conference should address itself to the question "What are my goals and objectives?"; evaluation should help to answer personal self-development needs; different plans should be permitted for different departments, rather than insisting upon one hospital-wide evaluation plan; the evaluation process responsibilities and leadership requirements; head nurses should maintain on their own units the necessary records for evaluation purposes; review dates for evaluation sessions should be staggered to avoid having many persons scheduled for review within a few weeks' time once per year; a simple grading scale should be used; different types of plans should be permitted for differing job levels; the evaluation sessions should elicit feelings, attitudes and understandings about the implementation of important nursing programs such as nursing audit, PONS and MBO; evaluations should help to identify employees who have aspirations for growth and who intend to remain with the hospital; evaluations should be carried out only by nurse managers who are intimately familiar with the work results of the person being evaluated; the evaluation forms should allow space for comments, examples, critical incidents, and follow-through plans; standards of performance should be established against which actual work performance will be judged. This example is only one of many to demonstrate that pragmatic head nurses not only have justifiable criticism of existing employee appraisal programs, but also have excellent suggestions for an improved type of plan which they believe they could use with more enthusiasm and success. In the instance cited, such a plan was instituted which included practically all of the features which they recommended. The performance evaluation plan described herein successfully meets these same criteria.

Our purpose in this chapter is to describe an effective results-oriented performance evaluation program (ROPEP) which more and more administrators, department heads, nurse managers and other supervisory personnel are using to: (1) Identify performance responsibilities, (2) Develop measurable indicators of satisfactory performance, (3) Encourage employees to self-evaluate their own work performance, (4) Provide an objective basis for justifiable praise for creditable performance, (5) Assist employees in identifying their own needs for additional knowledge and skill, (6) Help employees to achieve maximum satisfaction from their work; and, when they so desire, to qualify themselves for jobs of greater responsibility.

INTRODUCTION TO PERFORMANCE EVALUATION

The term "performance evaluation" carries different meanings to different people. This is to be expected, since people's interpretation of a work-related word or phrase is based upon their own individual work experiences and the management techniques or personnel appraisal methods used in their places of employment. Performance evaluation as used in connection with ROPEP is defined as the measurement of the results of a person's work effort compared with previously agreed-upon standards of performance. This definition is broad enough to apply to the employee performance evaluation process at all job levels in every type of organization. It is specific enough to differentiate it from the variety of other terms used, sometimes erroneously, as synonyms.

Zollitsch and Langsner, devoting over 92 pages to "Fundamentals of Employee Evaluation" in their book *Wage and Salary Administration,* found over 70 different titles and descriptive terms used in connection with the evaluation of employees.[1] These terms included performance rating, appraisal and development rating, merit rating, efficiency rating, measuring performance, worker appraisal and performance review. What's in a name? A great deal! Does it make any difference what name is used to describe the technique? Yes! It makes a difference because of the unfavorable experiences of employees who have been subjected to or required to use so many of the poorly designed or ineffectively applied rating systems in the past.

The focus of many rating or appraisal methods has been on characteristics of the employee rather than upon the employee's demonstrated performance results. In fact, too many hospitals and other healthcare agencies still use appraisal forms that require supervisors to "measure" such factors as initiative, loyalty, cooperativeness, creativity, dependability, stamina, appearance, personality, potential, or interpersonal relations. The use of these kinds of characteristics for rating purposes causes unnecessary resentments, diverts attention from more meaningful objective measures of work results, subverts the laudable goals of the evaluation process and often contributes to making the entire program a matter of ridicule and scorn by both hourly paid employees and managers.

Abe Lincoln's oft-quoted statement is relevant here: "I do the very best I know how — the very best I can; and I mean to keep doing so until the end. If the end brings me out all right, what is said against me won't amount to anything. If the end brings me out wrong, ten angels swearing I was right would make no difference."[2] We believe that these words of Abe Lincoln express succinctly the attitudes of the great bulk of the thousands of healthcare employees with whom we have worked. We believe that these workers at all levels deserve evaluation methods that treat them more like adults than as children, and that give recognition to their common sense, worth as individuals, and human needs.

Some further clarification of terminology should be helpful before the results- oriented performance evaluation approach is presented. Such clarification will help to avoid later confusion and misunderstandings. "Job Evaluation" is the management technique for determining the relative worth of individual jobs in an organization so as to establish a wage classification system for that organization. "Employee Evaluation", sometimes called merit rating, is the subjective process of appraising the relative worth of employees to the organization in terms of their abilities, job performance and potential. Thus while job evaluation measures the relative worth of jobs, employee evaluation measures the relative worth of employees.

Theoretically, therefore, when both techniques are used effectively the amount of each employee's pay is determined by the worth of his job together with the measure of his own individual worth. Such a method attempts to provide equitable pay for persons doing the same or different jobs.

For example, the pay range for the LPN I classification may be $3.00 to $3.20 per hour (based upon job evaluation). Sue Smith, LPN, may be receiving $3.05 per hour while Alice Atwood, LPN, is paid $3.10 per hour (based upon their individual employee evaluations). Similarly, two persons who work in the LPN II classification of $3.20 to $3.50 per hour (based upon job evaluation) may be receiving the same pay of $3.30 per hour if they have the same relative worth as individuals (determined by employee evaluation). At the same time these LPN II's may have merit ratings equal to Alice Atwood, the LPN I, as judged on the employee evaluation scale.

OTHER FACTORS INFLUENCING WAGES

From a practical standpoint, a variety of other factors have a great influence upon the actual wages and salaries paid to individuals. Such factors include length of service, supply and demand, competition, ability to pay (financial conditions), wage and price controls, labor unions, philosophy of the organization as interpreted by management, personal preferences, fringe-benefits package, and current goals and priorities of the organization. In the final analysis, techniques such as job evaluation and employee evaluation are methods for assisting managers in establishing a fair day's pay for a fair day's work. They help to narrow the range of judgement within which a manager has to make decisions affecting each employee's pay. To this extent, these techniques and others like them can be useful.

Some organizations, however, have adopted a policy of

disassociating employee evaluation from the process of setting wage rates and salaries for individuals. This is in recognition and acceptance of the influence of the aforementioned factors that dictate what changes occur in wage payments from year to year. Such a policy has the advantage of permitting the employee evaluation process to take place in an atmosphere free of the concerns related to pay adjustments. The major focus of attention can then be the performance of the employee in carrying out his job duties and responsibilities, and how the employee and his own manager evaluate the performance results.

ROPEP DEFINITION CLARIFIED

ROPEP is an effective method for the evaluation of performance results. The key words in the definition of performance evaluation (as previously stated in this chapter) can now be examined for their meaning in the light of the prior discussion. *Performance evaluation* is the *measurement* (the determination of degree of conformity with criteria of quality and quantity) of the *results* (consequences, outcomes) of a person's *work effort* (on- the- job activities and exertion) *compared* (examined in order to note the similarities or differences) with previously *agreed upon* (jointly developed in advance with accord by the manager and the employee) *standards* (acknowledged measures of comparison for qualitative or quantitative value; criteria; norms).

The following sections of this chapter describe the several phases of introducing and implementing ROPEP so that performance evaluation, as defined and clarified above, may become a reality. The four necessary phases are as follows: Phase 1, Preparing Performance Descriptions; Phase 2, Initial Application; Phase 3, The First Evaluation Cycle; and Phase 4, The Work Evaluation Cycle.

PHASE 1: PREPARING PERFORMANCE DESCRIPTIONS

A performance description has some similarities to a job description, but the two are basically different because they are developed for two different purposes. The job description, by its very title, describes a job. It is prepared by a process of job analysis. Its purpose is primarily to provide the necessary descriptive job information for job evaluation. A performance description, by contrast, describes performance responsibilities. It is prepared by a process of performance analysis carried out by employees with their own managers (supervisors, department heads, bosses). Its purpose is to reach agreement and understanding, between employee and manager, regarding the employee's performance responsibilities so that meaningful, ongoing self-evaluation of performance can take place.

A performance description is defined as a statement of the purpose of a person's job functions, the major performance responsibilities (grouped by persons to whom the responsibilities exist), and measures of satisfactory performance. The emphasis in the preparation of a performance description is upon reaching a mutual understanding between employee and manager regarding who is to do what for whom, when, and how well; so that there can be later understanding and agreement regarding what was done for whom, when, and how well. When an organization, a department, or an individual manager decides to use the ROPEP method, the essential first step is to prepare performance descriptions. This is a time consuming but rewarding process. This section describes how to do it.

ROPEP requires performance descriptions, not job descriptions. Do not make the mistake of attempting to adapt existing job descriptions to the purposes of ROPEP. To do so is to risk the success of the entire program since the performance descriptions and the process of preparing them provide the foundation upon which everything else is built.

Prior discussion has already emphasized that performance descriptions are the outcome of the combined efforts of each manager and the employees who work for that manager. The process of coming together to discuss the performance responsibilities and the measures of satisfactory performance and of reaching mutual understanding and agreement regarding them is even more important than the actual wording of the statements that become the written form of the performance descriptions. Once understanding is achieved, the interpretation of the words and the meanings of the performance descriptions is likely to be uniform. Lacking such mutual understanding, agreement upon the other phases of the performance evaluation process becomes much more difficult.

One of the best ways for two persons to reach an understanding is for them to talk together fully and openly. When the two persons involved are a nurse manager and a staff member, it is necessarily the manager who must set the example and create the climate for such open discussion. An essential element is the manager's ability to draw out the employee's views with suitable questions, then to listen carefully to what the employee says. This is a skill too often poorly developed by some managers. Listening is difficult; listening takes time; listening is hard work; listening is tiring. Listening skill is essential, however, and it can be developed.

Performance Description Worksheet

Another important way to involve personnel as a part of the process of securing understanding regarding performance requirements is the use of a Performance Description Worksheet. A sample of such a worksheet is included in Appendix D. This type of worksheet to be completed by every employee in every job provides for valuable input by the people who know the most about their performance responsibilities—namely, the people doing the work. When all of the responses from all of the employees with the same job title are summarized, a wealth of information is available for preparing a meaningful first draft of the major performance responsibilities for that particular job—as described by the employees themselves. Similarly, some excellent clues to suitable measures of satisfactory performance are provided by employee responses to the question, "How do you know when you are doing a good job?"

The Performance Description Worksheets can be distributed by nurse managers at small departmental or unit meetings. Appropriate explanations of the purpose of the worksheets can then be given, with time for questions and answers. It is helpful to state the purpose of the worksheets, with instructions for completing them, directly on the worksheet forms. This will minimize misunderstandings and concerns regarding their purpose.

Should these worksheets be signed or should they be completed anonymously? We believe they should be signed. To do otherwise is to start off on the wrong foot with a program designed to strengthen the most important of all on-the-job relationships—that between employees and managers. Anonymous questionnaires smack too much of the kind of gameplaying that ROPEP seeks to eliminate. Admittedly there may be some organizational circumstances that dictate unsigned responses when the worksheets are used for the first time. Whenever this is the case, it is symptomatic of significant administrative, supervisory or labor relations problems that deserve attention before ROPEP is introduced.

As with PONS and MBO, the introduction of an important technique such as ROPEP often is long delayed, awaiting a top-level administrative exploration, decision and implementation effort. This is unfortunate, because more often than not there is no need for a uniform plan to be used agency-wide. In fact, there may be valid reasons for using varied approaches, different starting dates and different implementation steps for such techniques within different departments of a hospital. With this in mind, we provide in the Appendix D some guidelines and specific implementation steps which can be used by nurse managers independently within their own areas of responsibility. The steps are remarkably simple. They make sense to nurse managers who have followed them. All that you need in order to do the same thing yourself are some of the characteristics of being a nurse manager previously discussed: motive force, willingness to take some reasonable risks, ability to use the Decision Worksheet, a sense of agreement with McGregor's Theory Y and Myers' enriched job concept, and a desire to follow the simple instructions.

The approach, as you will see in Appendix D, is first of all to prepare your own performance description. The fact that you take the initiative (instead of your boss doing so) makes no difference. The more to your credit! It is important, however, that you seek the involvement of your boss. Both you and your boss need to agree upon what you should be doing for whom, when and how well. Then when you want an answer to the question, "How am I doing?", both you and your boss will be evaluating the same things by the same standards of satisfactory performance.

The Complete Performance Description

Appendix G provides an example of a performance description for a head nurse. An example of a performance description for a staff nurse position (RNII) as developed by nurse managers in one hospital may be found in Appendix D. The content of this description includes the position title and department name, titles of the employees supervised by the RN and a brief statement of the purpose (or primary function) of the nurse classified as RN II. Then the performance responsibilities and the measures of satisfactory performance are presented in a two-column format, as follows:

MAJOR PERFORMANCE RESPONSIBILITIES	PERFORMANCE IS SATISFACTORY WHEN:
To Patients (or other agency clients)	(For each item, a statement is made of the measurable conditions which will exist when performance is satisfactory.)
To Medical Staff	
To Own Nurse Manager	
To Unit Personnel	
To Committees	
To Other Department Personnel	
To Other Organizations	
To Self	

The major performance responsibilities listed are what the RN IIs in this hospital have to do in their work, . listed under the person or persons for whom the responsibilities are performed. In the right-hand column, opposite each item of major responsibility on the left side, is the statement of measurable conditions that will exist when performance is satisfactory. Each of these measures is a completion of the sentence beginning, "Performance is satisfactory when...." The final section of the performance description is a listing of the qualifications necessary to become an RN II as established for this hospital department of nursing service. The qualifications section may or may not be included as part of a performance description, depending upon the total purposes which the description is intended to serve. This section is useful when a wide-track careers program (with clearly defined career ladders) is being instituted to identify promotional opportunities within the organization and how to qualify for them.

PHASE 2: THE INITIAL APPLICATION

When nurse managers prepare to initiate their first ROPEP evaluations with their departmental employees, they will find that each employee is at a different stage of readiness for their evaluations. Those who have had the opportunity to participate in Phase 1 and have actively contributed to the development of their performance descriptions are likely to be the best prepared. Newer employees and others who for one reason or another were not able to participate directly in Phase 1 will be far less informed and will require the greatest amount of initial orientation to the first use of the performance descriptions for the self-evaluation procedure.

Exhibit 4:1 is a Manager's Guide and Checklist for the Use of Performance Descriptions in Role Clarification and Performance Evaluation—An Employee Self-Evaluation Method. The emphasis in the method described is upon self-evaluation of performance results by each employee. This is a necessary step. As Frederick Herzberg says: "A real method of instilling the potential of accountability is to remove the crutch of inspection and instead directly identify the performance of the work with the individual."[3] To do otherwise is to perpetuate the record of failure, friction and frustration that has been characteristic of traditional employee appraisal and performance review plans in so many healthcare organizations. Herewith is a detailed explanation of each step included in the guidesheet for the Employee Self-Evaluation Method.

Exhibit 4:1
Manager's Guide & Checklist for the Use of Performance Descriptions in Role Clarification and Performance Evaluation
An Employee Self-Evaluation Method

A.   Meet with each employee to discuss and reach a mutual understanding of the employee's responsibilities and measures of satisfactory performance.

    ________ 1.   Review the performance description.

    ________ 2.   Ask for comments and questions.

    ________ 3.   Clarify and amplify the performance description through discussion.

    ________ 4.   Explain the self-evaluation procedure (including the exception principle).

B.   Establish a plan for regular employee self-evaluation.

    ________ 1.   Set a date for completion of first self-evaluation.

    ________ 2.   Obtain from employees their own written comments regarding how well they think they are meeting each of their performance responsibilities. (The Self-Evaluation of Performance record may be used.)

C.   Meet with employees individually to review their self-evaluations.

    ________ 1.   Set dates for the discussions.

    ________ 2.   Meet with the employees individually and listen to their comments.

    ________ 3.   Agree whenever possible with the employee's own performance evaluation of the major performance responsibilities.

    ________ 4.   When you disagree with the self-evaluation of a responsibility, ask the employees to explain again their reasons for their own evaluation. Then indicate why you feel that the performance results are better than, or not as good as, the employee's own evaluation.

    ________ 5.   Reach agreement upon those performance results which need strengthening.

    ________ 6.   Develop suggestions for improvement with the employee. Help identify available resources.

    ________ 7.   Agree upon specific follow-through action.

Manager's Guide to Using Performance Descriptions

Here is an elaboration of each step outlined on the manager's guide and checklist (Exhibit 4:1).

A. Meet with each employee to discuss and reach a mutual understanding of the employee's performance responsibilities and measures of satisfactory performance.

1. Review the performance description.

This step is considerably simplified when the employee helped to prepare the statements in the performance description. When this is the case, there may be a temptation to omit this first step on the assumption that it is not necessary. Resist such a temptation. Circumstances change. Ongoing work experiences can change a person's viewpoints and interpretations. A person's apperceptive mass continues to evolve. So while this first step may take less time with the employee who was involved in the first writing of the performance description, include this step always with each and every employee as part of every periodic evaluation discussion.

2. Ask for comments and questions.

The intent in this step is to encourage an open, free and easy exploration of what the employee's work is all about—its purpose, what has to be done for whom, and so on. How each manager brings about this kind of discussion depends greatly upon the manager's own individual style. What works well for one person may not work so well for another. However, a vital factor that has a great influence upon the level of communication that takes place is the attitude that the manager brings to the discussion. This will be communicated and will influence what happens. Some tips for stimulating productive discussion are included in these pages.

3. Clarify and amplify the performance descriptions, through discussion.

This is especially essential for the first meeting with employees who have not previously seen the performance description for their jobs. This cannot be hurried. Whatever time it takes will be time well spent. (How long does it take and how much does it cost to process a grievance? A labor arbitration case? A lawsuit in court?) Ask repeatedly, "What does this mean to you?" Request, "Tell me in your own words what this means." Reiterate, "The reason we are doing this is so that both you and I have the same understanding about your work and what we can expect of each other." Say,

"What I think I heard you say was...(repeat what employee said). Do you mean that...(try to give same message in different words of your own choosing)?" Give an example to illustrate the meaning; say, "For example, if a patient asks to be helped out of bed, then slips and falls on the floor, do you mean that you would...(etc.)?"

4. Explain the self-evaluation procedure (including the exception principle).

The self-evaluation aspect of ROPEP is a theme that requires emphasis throughout every step of ROPEP. Explain, "The reason for our having this kind of a self-evaluation program is so that you can feel comfortable doing your work without having me looking over your shoulder. Most people don't like the idea of a manager being a 'snoopervisor.' I don't like it either. The best way for both of us to get along together is for us to understand what both of us (you and me) consider to be satisfactory performance of your responsibilities. So let's take a look at these again."

Explain that:

(a) The *first* regular performance evaluation discussion will include *all* of the performance responsibilities.

(b) Subsequent regular evaluations (once or twice per year) will focus on those performance results which are exceptionally outstanding or exceptional because they do not meet the standard of satisfactory performance. This is the exception principle. All other performance results require no attention because they are all satisfactory.

(c) Performance evaluation is really an ongoing day-to-day process. Thus there are likely to be many occasions between regular evaluation review sessions when the performance descriptions will need to be used to clarify questions, remind each other of performance standards, help to plan skill-improvement programs and for other work-related purposes.

B. Establish a plan for regular employee self-evaluation.

1. Set a date for completion of first self-evaluation.

A date for completing the first self-evaluation may be set during the foregoing discussion in Step A4. Much depends upon the readiness of the individual employees. One person may require more than one discussion to complete the steps A1 through A4. Another person may be ready to carry out his own self-evaluation immediately following step A4.

The manager will be able to judge how soon to allow the self-evaluation step to be completed. The manager can say, "How soon will you want to complete your first self-evaluation of performance?" There is usually no need to hurry it. For one person it may be within the month; for another, two or three months.

2. Obtain from employees their own written comments regarding how well they think they are meeting each of their performance responsibilities.

Remind employees to include every performance responsibility in this first self-evaluation. An extra copy of the performance description can be used by the employees on which to record their comments. For subsequent evaluations, the form in Fig. 4:3 can be used. Whatever form is used, the employee is expected to submit it to the manager by the date agreed upon.

Encourage employees to discuss with you (as manager) their efforts at self-evaluation if they wish to do so. They may need nothing more than to have some time with you to tell you how they are progressing, and to have you agree with the kinds of words they are using. This interchange prior to the actual evaluation discussion can be highly valuable in preparing both employee and manager for a productive follow through.

C. Meet with employees individually to review their self-evaluations.

1. Set dates for the discussions.

Establishing and maintaining a schedule for evaluation discussions is an indication of the importance attached to this activity by the nurse manager. Allow ample flexibility in the time planned for each individual evaluation discussion so that there will be no need to cut short a discussion that is proving to be lengthy but productive. It is good practice to schedule no more than one person for an evaluation session on any one day.

2. Meet with employees individually and listen to their comments.

Even when the manager has the employee's written self-evaluation comments in advance of the discussion, there is merit in permitting the employee to explain the self-evaluation verbally in the evaluation session. It is part of the process of maintaining a maximum level of communications and understanding at a most crucial point in the procedure.

3. Agree whenever possible with the employee's own performance evaluation of the major performance responsibilities.

The purpose of this procedure is to reach a meeting of minds (the manager's and the employee's) regarding the employee's performance results. Seek areas of agreement, not disagreement. The main question to be agreed upon for each performance responsibility is: "Has performance been satisfactory or not satisfactory, as measured against the stated criteria in the performance description?"

4. When you disagree with the self-evaluation of a responsibility, ask the employee to explain again the reasons for the evaluation. Then indicate why you feel that the performance results are better than or not as good as the employee's own evaluation.

If both the employee and the manager have the same understanding of the responsibilities being evaluated and of the measures of satisfactory performance, then any disagreement in an evaluation would stem from differing knowledge of actual performance results (or differing interpretations of those results). The process of examing each of these three aspects in turn for any performance responsibility on which there appears to be a lack of agreement will minimize the likelihood of unnecessary misunderstandings.

The manager should maintain adequate personnel records to provide factual back-up data for unsatisfactory performance as well as for exceptionally good performance. Such documentation is essential for a number of valid purposes related to accreditation standards, nursing audit, patient care, lawsuits, labor relations when unions are involved, and effective personnel administration. One of the useful documentation methods is the critical incident technique as described by Fivars and Gosnell in *Nursing Evaluation: The Problem and The Process.*[4]

5. Reach agreement upon those performance results which need strengthening.

This step is not always necessary with all employees for every regular performance evaluation. One of the fallacies connected with employee evaluation practices is the idea that there is always something wrong with employees or with their performance. Rating forms frequently seem to encourage emphasis on weaknesses rather than strengths. No wonder the appraisal procedure has such a bad reputation!

It is not necessary to make a special effort to find evidence of poor performance results that require improvement. Managers need not feel that they are poor evaluators if they cannot always identify weaknesses in employees' performances. On the contrary, managers should take credit when they have provided the kind of training and leadership which minimizes or eliminates the un-satisfactory performance results.

But when performance results have been less than satisfactory, they must be faced for what they are. Hopefully, both the manager and the employee will recognize and agree upon the evidence of un-satisfactory performance results. Whenever there is a lack of such agreement, and the manager is convinced that the results for a given major performance responsibility are clearly unsatisfactory, then he must make his own evaluation known to the employee and proceed in whatever manner is most likely to secure the satisfactory level of performance that is necessary.

6. Develop suggestions for improvement with the employee. Help identify available resources.

Here again, as for item #5, this is not always a necessary part of the self-evaluation process with all employees. Significant numbers of employees are likely to be delivering satisfactory performance for all of their major performance responsibilities. Many of this group of employees are valuable in their present jobs, have no need to im-prove their performance and have no desire to qualify for higher-paid positions. They form an important and usually stable portion of the workforce. They are using their assets well and deserve credit for doing so.

When improvement is required on one or more performance responsibilities, ask the employee, "What do you want to do about it?" If improvement is to occur, it has to come about through the ef-forts of the individual employees. They have to motivate themselves to make improved performance happen. The manager can suggest sources of help and guidance when it is wanted. When necessary, the manager can prescribe the remedy that appears to be needed to secure results.

7. Agree upon specific follow-through action.

This is the specific outcome of a regular performance self-evaluation discussion. This step answers the questions, "What happens now? What do we do next?" For some employees the follow-through is signified by a parting comment on the part of the manager, "Keep up the good work." For other employees there will be an understanding of agreed-upon action by the employee (and perhaps the manager also) that will lead to the correction of those performance results which have been unsatisfactory. This agreement should be in writing, and follow the general pattern of the management-by-objectives technique—set a goal; set a date;

evaluate. The objectives worksheet (found in Appendix D) provides a simple way to record this information for future follow-through.

The Meaning of Satisfactory Performance

There are some evident similarities between ROPEP and Nursing Audit as management techniques. Both are evaluative processes. Both establish standards of performance for measurement purposes. Both seek to provide criteria that will lead to employee performance results that assure the optimum delivery of patient care services. Both use a "go, no-go" concept of measurement (as discussed in Chapter 5).

The measure of satisfactory performance as used in connection with major performance responsibilities in patient care is a demanding standard. Thus the statement, "Performance is satisfactory when there are no documented errors," means no errors — none at all. There are few jobs in the world of work where such a stringent standard is required. But can anything else be "satisfactory" in any aspect of health care so vital, for example, as that of giving medications? Drucker makes the point nicely in writing about decision-making and the need for compromise in order to balance conflicting objectives, conflicting opinions and conflicting priorities.

> One has to compromise in the end. But unless one starts out with the closest one can come to the decision that will truly satisfy objective requirements, one ends up with the wrong compromise — the compromise that abandons essentials.

> For there are two different kinds of compromise. One kind is expressed in the old proverb 'Half a loaf is better than no bread .' The other kind is expressed in the story of the Judgment of Solomon, which was clearly based on the realization that "half a baby is worse than no baby at all." In the first instance, objective requirements are still being satisfied. The purpose of bread is to provide food, and half a loaf is still food. Half a baby, however, is not half of a living and growing child. It is a corpse in two pieces.[5]

PHASE 3: THE FIRST EVALUATION CYCLE

ROPEP may appear to be a detailed, time-consuming procedure. It is. But what are the alternatives? Other employee appraisal techniques are time consuming also and often generate results that are far

Figure 4:1

Management by Objectives for Nursing

A Graphic Outline of the ROPEP/MBO Procedure

The Nurse Manager's Job Responsibility

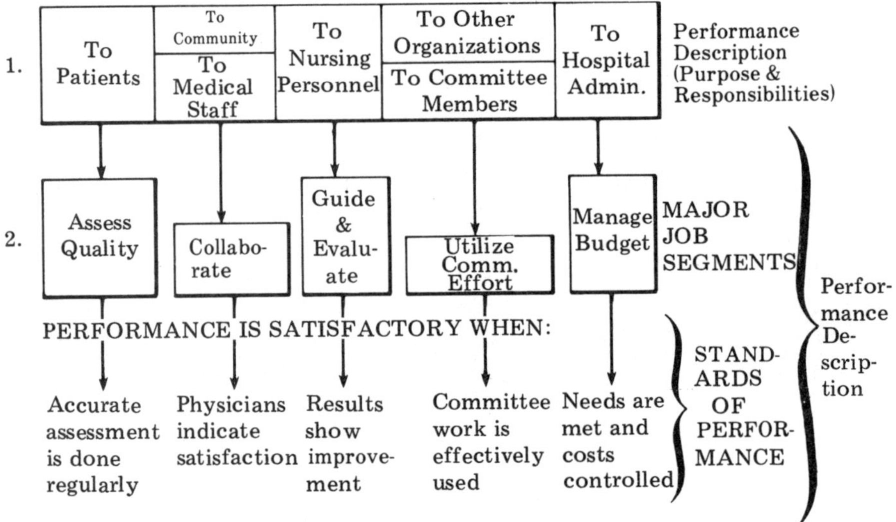

4. SET SPECIFIC GOALS

   Set Objective
   Set Target Dates

5. DO THE TASKS NECESSARY TO MEET THE SET OBJECTIVES

6. REVIEW PERFORMANCE ON SET TARGET DATE

   Set New and Revised Objectives
   Set New Target Dates

---

from satisfactory. ROPEP builds upon a combination of the human and technical modes in management that work well at all organizational levels. The focus is upon people doing the work of the organization— the needs, goals and performance of people as related to the needs, goals and performance of the organization. Thus ROPEP is an integral part of a management-by-objectives program within an organization.

Figure 4:1, entitled Management by Objectives for Nursing, summarizes in six steps the functioning of an integrated MBO System that uses performance descriptions as the basis for employee performance evaluation in relation to individual objectives within the pattern of the broad departmental and organizational goals. In the example, the position used is that of a nurse manager (head nurse, supervisor, patient care coordinator, assistant director of nursing service, etc.). The six steps of the ROPEP/MBO procedure are: (1) identify purpose and performance responsibilities (to whom); (2) list the major job segments (details of performance responsibilities); (3) develop measures of satisfactory performance; (4) set goals, objectives, and target dates; (5) work toward achievement of objectives; and (6) review performance results; plan new objectives and target dates.

The consistency of relationships between and the similarities of purpose for the various management techniques and the management functions are evident. Management techniques (by whatever name) are action plans, procedures or programs to assist nurse managers in using their skills to perform one or more management functions. The management techniques of ROPEP and MBO may be carried out in a variety of ways in different agencies and under a variety of names or without any identifying names at all. The merit in having a name to identify a worthwhile method or procedure is that it facilitates communications about it, minimizes misunderstandings, distinguishes it from other less satisfactory versions intended for the same purpose and helps in the training of newer nurse managers in the art and science of their profession.

Where to Begin

Organizations, like people, must start from where they are when they undertake a new learning or developmental program. Each is at a different state of readiness. Some hospitals have had considerable experience with one or more types of appraisal systems. Others have had little or none. Some organizations will want to adopt ROPEP as part of building a strong personnel program with effective manager—employee relations to minimize the likelihood of a union. Others will begin to use ROPEP *because* they have a union.

But while there may be variations in how to begin to implement ROPEP, a sound practice is to begin always with the administrative and management group first. No managers at any level should be expected to carry out any of the ROPEP steps with employees under their direction until they have been on the receiving end of the process themselves. Is this dictum idealistic? Yes! Is it too idealistic for most healthcare agencies? No! One of the reasons for the failure of appraisal systems generally is that administrators and chief executives have approved the installation of such systems for use by middle managers with lower-echelon employees without having been willing to implement the plan with the people that work directly for them. Had they done so, many of these appraisal plans would have been abandoned before they were exposed to the justified disdain of managers at lower organizational levels. ROPEP should not be introduced into a hospital whenever the administrator or chief executive is unwilling to use ROPEP first with those persons who report directly to him or her. This admonition should be heeded for a number of reasons:

- Top administrative and middle management personnel require effective evaluation of their own performance for the same reasons as do others in the organization. The suitable use of ROPEP at the higher organizational levels is even more essential than at lower levels because of the greater impact of satisfactory or unsatisfactory individual performance of top-level managers upon organizational goal achievement.
- The critical, analytical use of ROPEP by top administrators will contribute to whatever adaptations may be necessary for its most effective ongoing use within that hospital or agency.
- Managers learn by doing, just the same as other people. Part of the learning process is to carry out all of the steps of ROPEP "for real," including developing the measures of satisfactory performance, self-evaluation, and follow-through of the MBO cycle.
- ROPEP gains in credibility, just as does any other technique, when the manager can say to employees with conviction, "This is not just for you. My boss uses it with me too."
- There isn't any other successful way to do it. Review the ROPEP-MBO cycle as part of your management functions. It will be obvious that the suggested approach for using ROPEP does not add work. It simply helps to organize and systematize the already essential elements of the manager's performance responsibilities—at all levels.

Steps B1 and 2, and steps C1 through 7, of the Manager's Guide and Checklist for ROPEP (as shown in Figure 4:1 and the accompanying description) present a way to plan and carry out the initial self-evaluation with employees when ROPEP is just beginning. Subsequent self-evaluation discussions follow easily at appropriate intervals, and will require less total time than the first series of evaluations using the two-column performance descriptions as the results-oriented basis for measurement. As the process continues through several evaluation cycles over the first year or two, the exciting benefits of ROPEP will become apparent as an essential basic technique in the nurse manager's repertoire.

PHASE 4: THE WORK EVALUATION CYCLE

Much emphasis has been placed upon the mutual development of performance descriptions which represent an understanding between employee and manager regarding who is to do what for whom, when, and how well. These same elements of performance were used as the basis for the self-evaluation procedure that has been described.

The early phases of setting up and initiating ROPEP are necessary for a successful performance evaluation program. This is true for any management technique—the preparation and beginning phases are more time consuming than the ongoing use and maintenance of the program. Yet suitable help and guidance can minimize the time requirements for introducing the program and completing the performance descriptions. An additional benefit of such help is the training of the management personnel who will coordinate the program and serve as organizational resource persons.

The six steps of the ROPEP-MBO cycles (Figures 3:5 and 4:1) demonstrate how the performance evaluation concept is broadened to include all aspects of a person's performance goals—the regular job performance responsibilities as well as those periodically assigned performance objectives. The latter are a natural outgrowth of the ROPEP method since some objectives will relate to necessary action needed to secure a satisfactory level of performance for one or more major performance responsibilities. There is a danger, however, in placing overemphasis upon identifying and attempting to correct deficiencies. Certainly errors and grossly unsatisfactory performance cannot be allowed to continue. But the focus needs to be upon identifying the *strengths* of individuals and in building upon these strengths for the benefit of all. To do otherwise is to ignore the findings of motivational research as well as to blind ourselves to the meaning of the life/work experiences of each one of us.

This section considers the ongoing, continuous evaluation process once the initial developmental stages of ROPEP have been completed and the first self-evaluation cycle has occurred. An important reminder is that ROPEP is *not* a once-a-year enforced appraisal routine scheduled to coincide with the "annual merit increase." This phrase is one often used, tongue-in-cheek, by those who recognize the hypocrisy of the term "merit" for a wage adjustment process that is influenced primarily by a variety of other factors as described early in this chapter.

More often than not the governing principle that appears to dictate wage adjustments is: "Every employee worth keeping is worth paying as high an across-the-board general increase as we can afford." Such a policy is understandable in these times of major financial stress due to inflation and the increasing restraints imposed by union contracts and consumer or government-inspired wage and price controls. Such a principle *implies* performance evaluation in the phrase "worth keeping." Some employees may not justify an increase in wages based upon their performance. But they receive the increase nonetheless. Some of them by any objective measure should have been dropped from the hospital payroll years ago. These are the "touchy" cases that require special attention and action. In any event, the sham and cost of an annual formal personnel appraisal in the traditional mode is unnecessary to justify the nickel-and-dime "merit" wage adjustments that have been so typical.

While ROPEP will assist meaningfully in the annual wage adjustment decisions, this is not its primary purpose. Its principal purpose is to provide a technique and the tools to assist nurse managers in getting people to do well what has to be done because *they* want to do it.

The Day-to-Day Use of ROPEP and MBO

The point has been made previously that an effective performance evaluation procedure is not an "add-on" to a manager's regular workload. More accurately, ROPEP and MBO become an integral part of the manager's three main functions: planning, doing, controlling. Compare the three management functions with the three steps of ROPEP and of MBO. These are summarized on page 129.

These cyclical processes are going on daily in one form or another for managers and other employees alike. They are never ending. They are mutually dependent and supportive. They are this way because they are based upon proven principles and practices of participation and involvement of people working together toward common objectives. When ROPEP and MBO are seen as month-in and month-out,

ROPEP CYCLE	MANAGEMENT FUNCTIONS CYCLE	MBO CYCLE
Perform Job Segments	DO	Perform Necessary Work
Identify Performance Responsibilities and Standards	PLAN	Set Goals and Objectives
Measure Performance Against Standards	CONTROL	Review Progress (was objective achieved on time?)

year-round ways of managing, the occasions for discussing self-evaluations of performance are many. These occur naturally in the course of a day's work and by plan when needed. Effective managers know that evaluation discussions are most worthwhile when they occur soon after the specific performance results that drew attention.

The more formal semiannual or annual general reviews using the complete performance descriptions can be scheduled if desired. But these need not be grouped together in one month of the year. Like the billings for renewals of magazine subscriptions or for automobile drivers' licenses, they can be scheduled to spread the workload throughout the year by using employment anniversary dates, birth dates or a similar method.

Insofar as individual performance goals and objectives are concerned, they too are always in varying stages of identification, initiation, effecting and completion. Even when MBO objectives are related to budgetary planning, as is often the case, an effective ABP (annual budgetary planning) program will minimize an excessive concentration of objectives-related effort in any one month.

ROPEP: A Program Performance Plan

Figure 4:2 provides a summary of the four phases of introducing ROPEP. This program performance plan is so designed that it can

Figure 4:2

R O P E P
Results-Oriented Performance Evaluation Program
PROGRAM PERFORMANCE PLAN AND WORKSHEET
SCHEDULE BY MONTHS
PHASE 1
Develop Recommendation and plan
Secure Approval
Form ROPEP committee
Obtain input from employees (Complete performance description worksheet.)
Meet with groups of employees in each job category
Develop performance descriptions
Supplement with task lists as necessary
Determine wide-track career qualification requirement for each job level
PHASE 2
Introduce performance descriptions
Conduct inservice education programs on ROPEP
Establish ROPEP as part of orientation programs for all job levels
Achieve mutual understanding between nurse manager and nursing staff members about:
(1) Performance expectations
(2) When performance is satisfactory (Stds. of performance)
(3) Self-evaluation of performance
PHASE 3
Work performance period for all personnel
(3-6 months)
PHASE 4
Begin Self-evaluation of individual performance
Each person submits own self-evaluation form
Nurse manager reviews form and prepares for first self-evaluation interview
Conduct first round of self-evaluation interviews
Identify areas of mutual agreement on satisfactory and unsatisfactory performance
Set mutual objectives and dates for progress review
Day-to-day observation and coaching
Second round of self-evaluation interviews
ONGOING PROCESS
Annual self-evaluation reviews

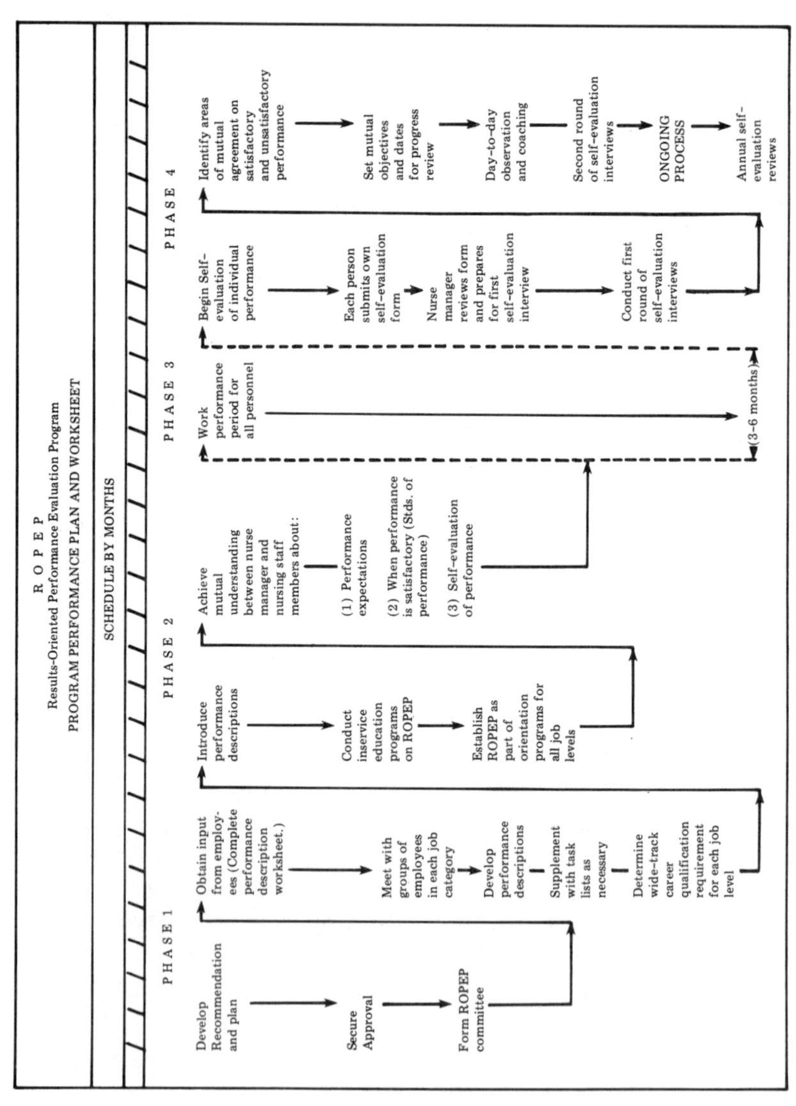

serve as a worksheet to assist you and others who may wish to introduce the ROPEP concept in your own agency or department. The program worksheet is intended to provide a flexible guide which can be adapted to your own situation with its unique organizational interrelationships, level of receptivity to newer management methods and timetable requirements.

The Systems Syndrome

Crystal balls went out of style years ago as part of the manager's tool kit. In actuality they never worked much better than Ouija boards. Hunches, sixth sense and feelings about situations and people have been more reliable when recognized for what they are and checked out accordingly. But managers tend to continue looking for a magic formula to help them do what they have to do — manage.

The trend toward the installation of and reliance upon systems is one manifestation of this understandable desire of managers to simplify their work of planning, doing and controlling. Systems are necessary. But they are no better than the persons who use them and manage them. Experience has demonstrated that well-motivated personnel using a poorly designed system ("no system at all") can achieve better performance results than poorly motivated personnel with a far more sophisticated system.

Some of the reasons for this phenomenon of motivated performance are set forth clearly in the writings of Douglas McGregor, Abraham Maslow, Peter Drucker, Frank Goble, and similar researchers and observers of people at work. Their message is clear. It is what effective managers have discovered repeatedly for themselves. This is the fact that managers cannot *make* employees give top performance results. Only the employees can *make themselves* give their best performance. If there is any kind of a crystal ball insight, a magic formula for managers, it lies in the awareness of this simple truth and how to create the motivational climate that permits employees to do their best. Some clues are provided herein, and in a later chapter.

Satisfactory vs. Top Performance

Why does ROPEP use measures of *satisfactory* performance instead of some higher goal of excellence? Perhaps the reasons are already evident. They include:

—ROPEP intends to be realistic in regard to what level of performance should be expected as a "fair day's work for a fair day's pay."

— The "satisfactory" standard is a demanding one, especially when the measure is "no errors" in the critical tasks of patient care.

— Managers and supervisors have learned through hard, frustrating experience the fallacies and hazards of more complicated appraisal methods.

— The *satisfactory* evaluation principle is consistent with labor-union philosophy and practice, as well as with sound personnel-administration policy.

— Excellence in performance often occurs in spite of, not because of, an appraisal program designed as a management control system to achieve it. Excellence is achieved by people with pride in their work, people who get satisfaction from their work.

This last reason is most significant. Certainly healthcare organizations need to strive for top performance and excellence today more than ever before. Competition, always a motivational factor in general-business organizations, is affecting hospitals and the healthcare industry too. Healthcare organizations must attract and hold as many people as possible who will do the work that has to be done—satisfactorily. ROPEP will help and contribute to creating a climate for top performance results.

Creating a Top-Performance Climate

Every organization, every department, tends to reflect the person at the head of it. That person's character, values and management concepts inevitably have a profound influence on creating the climate for performance that exists. Recognizing this, there is much that all nurse managers can do to affect the climate within which their people work and produce results. Tools, techniques and skills are necessary. Among these are communications skills that will help with the success of a program such as ROPEP.

It remains our conviction, however, that the character, values and attitudes of the nurse manager are paramount to successful performance. The nurse manager is the role model who trains, leads and evaluates the unit team workers who provide the level of care received by the patients. The challenge and responsibility are great. The rewards for satisfactory performance are highly personal and gratifying.

Later chapters include a variety of items that can be of assistance to managers who are attempting to implement ROPEP, MBO and other management techniques. The emphasis in these aids is not on systems and techniques in the traditional framework of management control. They stress a way of thinking about management and a set of value concepts that give balance to both the human mode and the technical mode. They are implicit in the following ROPEP Precepts:

1. Criticism has a negative effect on achievement of goals.
2. Honest appreciation has a positive effect on motivation.
3. Performance improves most when specific achievable goals are established.
4. Defensiveness resulting from a negative appraisal produces inferior performance.
5. Coaching should be a day-to-day, not a once-a-year, activity.
6. Mutual goal setting, not criticism, improves performance.
7. Interviews designed primarily for performance review purposes should not at the same time weigh in the balance a person's potential for salary increase or promotion.
8. Participation by employees in the objective-setting procedure helps produce favorable results.
9. In summary, compare the old review methods with the new results-oriented review procedure:

Focus of Old Review Methods	vs.	Focus of New Results-Oriented Review Methods
1. Personality	vs.	Specific goals and objectives
2. Weaknesses	vs.	Strengths (limited criticsm)
3. Unilateral goal setting	vs.	Mutual goal setting
4. Annual review	vs.	Day-to-day coaching
5. Looking back	vs.	Looking to future

As Frank Goble has said: "Workers are more perceptive than most managers realize. Whether their formal education is high or low, workers quickly see through managers who try to exploit and deceive them. It is essential that people within an organization receive fair treatment. When justice prevails, it is important that workers know it....Hand in hand with the need for justice is the need for a climate of trust. Unless this exists, all motivational attempts will fall far short of their full potential."[6]

NOTES

1. H. G. Zollitsch and A. Langsner, *Wage and Salary Administration* (Cincinnati: South- Western Publishing Co., 1970), p. 362.
2. Attributed to President Lincoln in a conversation with his Secretary of State, William H. Seward.
3. Frederick Herzberg, "The Wise Old Turk," *Harvard Business Review,* 52 (September- October 1974), p. 74.
4. Grace Fivars and Doris Gosnell, *Nursing Evaluation: The Problem and the Process* (New York: MacMillan, 1966), pp. 9-25.
5. Peter F. Drucker, *Management: Tasks, Responsibilities, Practices* (New York:Harper & Row, 1974), p. 479. Excerpt reprinted with permission.
6. Frank Goble, *Excellence in Leadership* (New York: American Management Association, 1972), p. 115.

SUGGESTED READINGS

Books

Carter, J.H.; Hilliard, M.; Castles, M.R.; Stoll, L.D.; and Cowan, A. *Standards of Nursing Care: A Guide for Evaluation,* 2nd ed., enlarged. (New York:Springer Publishing Co., 1976).

Drucker, Peter F. *The Effective Executive* (New York: Harper & Row, 1966.)

Drucker, Peter F. *Management: Tasks, Responsibilities, Practices* (New York: Harper & Row, 1974).

Fivars, Grace and Gosnell, Doris. *Nursing Evaluation: The Problem and the Process* (New York: MacMillan, 1966).

Ganong, Joan and Warren. *HELP with Management by Objectives* (Chapel Hill, N.C.: W.L. Ganong Co., 1975).

Ganong, Joan and Warren. *HELP with the Results- Oriented Performance Evaluation Program* (Chapel Hill, N.C.: W.L. Ganong Co., 1975).

Goble, Frank. *Excellence in Leadership* (New York: American Management Association, 1972).

Mager, R. F. *Analyzing Performance Problems* (Belmont, Calif.: Fearon Publishers, 1970).

Mager, Robert F. *Goal Analysis* (Belmont, Calif.: Fearon Publishers, 1972).

Marrow, Alfred. *The Failure of Success* (New York: Amacom, 1972).

Maslow, Abraham. *Eupsychian Management* (Homewood, Ill.: The Dorsey Press, 1965).

Maslow, Abraham. *Motivation and Personality* (New York: Harper & Row, 1970).

Maslow, Abraham. *Toward a Psychology of Being* (Princeton: Van Nostrand, Insight Books, 1968).

Morrison, George. *Management by Objective and Results* (Reading, Mass.: Addison-Wesley, 1970).

McGregor, Douglas. *The Human Side of Enterprise* (New York: McGraw-Hill, 1960).

Myers, M. Scott. *Every Employee a Manager: More Meaningful Work through Job Enrichment* (New York: McGraw-Hill, 1970).

Odiorne, George. *Management Decision by Objectives* (Englewood Cliffs, N.J.: Prentice-Hall, 1969).

Odiorne, George. *Management by Objectives* (New York: Pitman Publishing, Co., 1965).

Zollitsch, H.G. and Langsner, A. *Wage and Salary Administration* (Cincinnati, Ohio: South-Western Publishing Co., 1970).

Articles

Brady, Rodney, "MBO Goes to Work in the Public Sector," *Journal of Nursing Administration,* 3 (July-August 1973), p. 44.

Crowder, Dean and Bennett, Addison, "Total Commitment to Goals Is Secret of Hospital's Success," *Hospitals,* 50 (July 1, 1976), pp. 104-109.

Douglas, John et al., "A Progression Training Approach to Management by Objectives," *Training and Development Journal,* 27 (September, 1973).

Garant, Carol, "A Basis for Care," *American Journal of Nursing,* 72, (April 1972), pp. 699-701.

Hayes, James L., "How Am I Doing? Standards Tell," *Modern Healthcare,* 4 (August, 1975), p. 61.

Herzberg, Frederick, "The Wise Old Turk," *Harvard Business Review,* 52 (September-October 1974), pp. 70-80.

McConkey, Dale D. "Applying Management by Objectives to Non-Profit Organizations," *S.A.M. Advanced Management Journal,* 38 (January 1973), pp. 10-20.

McGregor, Douglas, "An Uneasy Look at Performance Appraisal," *Harvard Business Review,* 35 (May-June 1957), pp. 89-94.

Moore, Marjorie A., "Philosophy, Purpose, and Objectives: Why Do

We Have Them?" *Journal of Nursing Administration,* 1 (May-June, 1971), pp. 9-14.

Nuckolls, Katherine B., "Who Decides What the Nurse Can Do?" *Nursing Outlook,* 22 (October 1974), pp. 626-631.

Palmer, Jeanne, "Management by Objectives," *Journal of Nursing Administration,* 1 (January 1971), pp. 17-23.

Chapter 5
Nursing Audit and Quality Assurance

AUDIT, QUALITY AND ACCOUNTABILITY

Every healthcare agency needs to evaluate the quality of care patients receive and the quality of performance of the nursing staff. The entire concept of accountability in nursing rests on the ability to demonstrate the nature and quality of performance delivered by nursing personnel. The need for such accountability is dramatized by the rising cost of care without an equivalent rise in quality — or proof of that quality. The nurse manager has available a variety of management techniques to assist in delivering and evaluating the quality level of patient care. One of these techniques is the nursing audit. Nursing audit is, first of all, a method for assuring documentation of the quality of nursing care in keeping with the standards established by the agency, the nursing department and the professional, governmental and accrediting groups. Nursing audit is, therefore, part of the nurse manager's function of controlling, the third element in the three-phase management process.

As with other techniques, auditing works best when it is used as part of an integrated system — such as PONS. One of the strengths of the problem-oriented nursing system is its emphasis on assuring that patient needs and problems are identified and met with an appropriate level of care which is reflected accurately in the nursing audit results as reported.

Nursing audit provides the inspection method that compares results with the predetermined standards and criteria. As this inspection method is refined and improved, it measures more accurately than earlier practices the quality of the documentation of nursing care. Experience in every field of human endeavor indicates that when quality and performance standards (i.e., value considerations) are established, with results being measured against such standards, the results improve. There is increasing evidence that nursing audit helps to improve nursing results.

The guidelines for nursing audit take into account the variables among healthcare agencies and their relative performance capabilities. Every agency is expected to adapt to its own uses the fundamental philosophy and basic steps of nursing audit so that demonstrable progress and improvement can be achieved. It should be noted, however, that nursing audit is no cure-all. Documenting the level of quality that is delivered will not, in and of itself, improve the quality of care. You cannot inspect quality into a service; quality must be built into the service. In healthcare agencies the level of quality is determined at the point of service during all four phases of the nursing process. But audit certainly raises the level of awareness of the need for accurate and concise documentation in order to "prove" the care that has been given and the progress of the patient as the result of that care. Nurses must document, in the patient record, their contribution to helping resolve the identified needs and problems of patients and their families.

Management techniques alone cannot improve the quality of care. People improve quality through their use of techniques and skills and no technique is ever any better than the skills of the person using that technique. This is as true for nursing audit as it is for other management and clinical techniques. Nurses are among the people who provide services to, for and with patients and their families. Therefore nurses determine the quality level of the care being provided. But the patient is the one who experiences (feels, knows) the quality of care being received. And whatever the level of care may be, as experienced by the patient and his family, it deserves to be reflected as accurately as possible in the audit results. The purposes and benefits of nursing audit were discussed in Chapter 2 as a vital component of PONS. Our purpose now is to present sufficient details of the nursing audit procedure so that it can be understood as a useful nursing management technique.

ORGANIZING FOR NURSING AUDIT

Nursing audit has become mandatory for three basic reasons: the increasing cost of care; the need to improve quality of care; and the need for proof of the quality of care actually delivered—for yourself, your agency, third-party payers and interested others. Costs, quality and accountability are all inextricably woven together in the minds of consumers. With little or no choice or control over these factors, consumers—frustrated and apprehensive—seek ways to relieve their concerns.

Nursing staff members also seek to relieve the causes of their own frustrations. There is ample evidence of individual motivation, as well as departmental and institutional motivation, to improve the auditing process. Now there is available a tested and refined audit technique; and there are urgent reasons to put it to work. Some of the reasons for an audit are implicit in the definition of the term. "Audit," as a noun means an examination, adjustment or correction of records or accounts; as a verb, "audit" means to examine, verify, or correct (accounts, records, or claims). The implications for nursing personnel are clear; it is not adequate simply to provide satisfactory patient care. Such care must be fully documented as part of the patient's record.

The Joint Commission on Accreditation of Hospitals (JCAH) has summarized the basic requirements for audit. The hospital governing body has ultimate responsibility for the quality of care. The governing body delegates the evaluation of patient care provided by physicians to the medical staff and delegates the evaluation of patient care provided by others—nurses and allied health professionals—to administration. The medical and nursing staffs can use any organizational method they choose to accomplish audit. The audit procedure should include the following six steps:

1. Standards and criteria established.
2. Measurement of actual practice against criteria.
3. Evaluation of results.
4. Action taken to correct deficiencies.
5. Follow up and reassessment.
6. Report to nursing service, administration and medical staff.

The nursing administrator, as the delegate of the hospital administrator, has the responsibility to: (1) initiate and maintain a nursing audit program, (2) organize for audit using a method decided upon within nursing, (3) include the six basic steps in the audit procedure, and (4) evaluate all patient care services under the direction of the nursing department.

The first step in organizing a nursing audit program is establishing a nursing audit committee. The nursing administrator, in consultation with key personnel, establishes the committee with representation from the units and departments responsible for providing nursing care, maintaining records and unit management. The nursing audit committee may replace one or more existing committees or it may become a responsibility of an existing committee (such as the patient care committee). To make such a determination, the purposes and functions of existing committees must be compared with the purposes and functions of the audit committee.

This committee is charged with the initial task of developing guidelines for an audit program, setting clinical standards and criteria for measurement of results, deciding on forms, and performing the pilot audits to gain experience and test the instruments to be used. Following this preparatory work, the committee continues the ongoing process of guiding the planning, evaluating, recommending, teaching, communicating and corrective activities essential to the audit process.

The nursing audit program requires a considerable degree of cooperation between the medical records administrator, the nursing administrator and the audit committee. The responsibility of the medical records administrator does not include evaluating the adequacy of the nursing records nor their value in assisting the physician in his management of patient care. This responsibility lies with the audit committee and the nursing department. But the medical records administrator (or designee) is a valuable member of the audit committee. Once standards and criteria have been established the medical records department can do the retrieval of data needed for the nursing audit committee to evaluate the findings.

The nursing audit committee should be a standing committee of the department of nursing and should submit monthly and annual reports to the nursing administrator. Actual audits may be performed by personnel within specialty areas (i.e., medicine, surgery, obstetrics, pediatrics, psychiatry, cardiap care, emergency care, etc.) or by representatives from these specialties serving on the standing committee. Larger agencies may decentralize the auditing to subcommittees.

Membership of the audit committee should include representatives of all levels of professional nurses including patient care coordinators, supervisors, head nurses, staff nurses, clinical specialists and nurse clinicians. The chairman should be appointed, selected by the group, or designated based upon performance responsibilities and job title. Where applicable, licensed practical nurses, nursing assistants and other types of patient care personnel may be members of the audit committee. The medical records administrator (or designee) should be a regular member of the committee.

The functions of the audit committee may be summarized in two phases. During the first phase, when just established, the committee meets regularly to develop purposes and objectives; establish standards and criteria; establish guidelines for conducting audits; decide upon the necessary forms (using JCAH forms or adapting other forms to your needs); initiate the auditing process; practice auditing to become proficient; keep brief, pertinent minutes of all audit committee meetings including date, place, time, names of members (and guests) present, topics discussed, action agreed upon, recommendations and progress on previous recommendations. The second phase begins the actual implementation and maintenance of the audit procedure. The ongoing responsibilities of the committee include:

1. Plan audit sessions and schedule on a monthly basis (or periodically as required) to accomplish goals and objectives.
2. Arrange for Medical Records to pull charts for retrospective (closed chart) audits and retrieve data.
3. Evaluate audit results in committee.
4. Conduct quality control checks by observing direct nursing care; interviewing patients and personnel; auditing closed and open patient records, and other nursing records.
5. Prepare summaries of all audits and quality control checks for use by the nursing department and patient care units, and to serve as a report to hospital administration. JCAH requires that copies of such summaries be sent to the director of nursing, chief of the medical staff and to the board of trustees via the hospital administrator.
6. Teach professional nursing personnel the auditing process so they can become involved and share audit results with all nursing personnel.
7. Assist nursing personnel to utilize audit results to improve care and the documentation of care.
8. Make recommendations to appropriate hospital and nursing committees for policies, procedures, systems, services and materials or equipment that can improve care.
9. Keep brief, pertinent minutes of audit committee meetings (as in the first phase).

When the nursing staff and the medical staff combine to form a single audit committee, the above functions can be incorporated into that committee's activities. In any case, cooperation between the medical and nursing staffs in auditing is important and needs to be encouraged.

WORKING COMMITTEES:

A Nursing Audit Committee on Every Unit

One example of a committee plan with many benefits provides for decentralizing the audit function to the patient care units. Table 5:1 shows the structure, membership, and relationships of the committees. On the patient care units the audit activity is carried out by the Unit Nursing Care Committees. The purpose of each nursing care committee is to plan, coordinate, measure and improve the 24-hour nursing care activities for each nursing unit and specialty department so that the delivery of patient care will be consistent with the objectives of the nursing unit, the department and the hospital for quality care. Members include, for each nursing unit and specialty department, the head nurse, days, as chairman; the head nurse (charge nurse), evenings; and the head nurse (charge nurse), nights. (For the specialty departments such as OR and ER, membership less will be modified to fit the existing situation.)

The purpose of each nursing care team is to involve nursing unit shift personnel in the effective delivery of patient care, through the use of the nursing process for each patient. Members include for each nursing unit and specialty department the shift head nurse as chairman and all other unit personnel on the shift: staff nurses, licensed practical nurses, nurse aides, orderlies and unit secretaries. Where regular nursing care teams have already been used effectively, they may be continued as the basis for this link in the committee network.

This type of committee structure provides for the meaningful involvement of nursing personnel in committee work. It facilitates the job enrichment concepts of Frederick Herzberg, M. Scott Myers, and others. Skillfully used, these concepts greatly enhance the likelihood of success with a nursing audit program and its contributions to optimum patient care.

STANDARDS AND CRITERIA

A standard is an acknowledged measure of comparison for quantitative or qualitative value, criterion, norm. A criterion is a standard, rule or test on which a judgement or decision can be based. It is essential to establish clinical audit criteria against which to measure patient

Table 5:1
Summary of Working Committees Membership

PERSONNEL TITLES (Other comparable titles may be substituted)	NAMES OF COMMITTEES					
	COORDINATING	SYSTEMS & PROCEDURES	EMPLOYEE NEEDS	STAFF DEVELOP-MENT	AUDIT/ NURSING CARE	NURSING CARE TEAMS
Dir. of Nsg. Serv./PCA	Ch.					
Assoc. Dir. of Nsg. Serv.	*				Ch.	
Asst. Dir. Nsg. Serv. Days	*	Ch.				
Asst. Dir. Nsg. Serv. Eve.	*		Ch.	*		
Asst. Dir. Nsg. Serv. Nite	*	*				
Coord. Inserv. Ed./	*	*		Ch.		
Staff Development						
Supervisor, Evenings		*	*			
Supervisor, Nights		*	*			
Hd. Nurse/Pt. Care Coord.		Rep.	Rep.	Rep.	*	Mgr.
Charge Nurse		Rep.	Rep.	Rep.	*	Mgr.
Staff/Primary Nurse		Rep.	Rep.	Rep.	*	*
Licensed Pract. Nurse		Rep.	Rep.	Rep.	*	*
Nurse Aide		Rep.	Rep.	Rep.	Rep.	*
Orderly		Rep.	Rep.	Rep.		*
Ward Clerk/Unit Sec.		Rep.	Rep.	Rep.		*

KEY: * = Regular member.   Rep. = Selected representative of group.
Ch. = Chairman.   Mgr. = Unit manager (add team leader as necessary).

This table is adapted from Warren and Joan Ganong, "Reducing Organizational Conflict Through Working Committees," *Journal of Nursing Administration*, 2 (January-February 1972), p. 12.

outcomes and the process used by the nursing staff. Establishing standards and criteria is an initial task for the nursing audit committee.

Careful choice of words and accurate use of audit terminology influence the levels of understanding and acceptance that an audit committee achieves. The following definitions will help to clarify key terms used in connection with nursing audit:

Retrospective: Referring to a review or contemplation of things in the past.

Closed Chart: The completed patient record for a discharged patient, in the custody of the medical records department.

Open Chart: The patient record for a patient still receiving care within the hospital or agency.

Retrospective (Closed Chart) Audit: An inspection of a closed chart to evaluate its documentary reliability, completeness and compliance with the standards for nursing care as established by the agency, the nursing department, and the professional, governmental and accrediting groups.

Quality Control Check: The inspection of the nursing process (as evidenced by the open chart, the patient and nursing personnel) to evaluate compliance with established standards of nursing care.

Outcome Audit: Identifies patient outcomes, satisfactory and unsatisfactory, and the patterns of nursing care that appear to be responsible.

Process Audit: A deeper probe of already recognized (or suspected) problems in the nursing care process.

Marion E. Nicholls in "Quality Control in Patient Care" provides a helpful explanation of outcome (ends) standards and process (means) standards:

Nursing care standards can be divided into ends and means standards. The ends standards are patient oriented; they describe the changes desired in a patient's physical status or behavior. The means standards are nurse oriented; they describe the activities and behavior designed to achieve the ends standards. Properly stated, nursing care objectives are the ends standards and the plan of care (or nursing orders) is the means standard. Although the ends and means standards are interrelated, different information about each is required to determine if they are being met. An ends standard requires information about the patient. A means standard calls for information about the nurse's performance. To be effective as standards, objectives and plans must meet three criteria. The statements must be understandable. They must be achievable in terms of the resources of the patient, the nurses, and the agency. And, if control is to be achieved, they must be measurable.[1]

Standards are established by and received from a variety of sources including federal, state and local units of government, licensing agencies, accrediting organizations (JCAH, NLN), professional organizations (ANA), trade associations (AHA), institutions (hospital, mental health center), departments (nursing, medicine), patient care unit (CCU, OR, psychiatric), and individuals (one's own personal standards). Standards, from whatever source and however developed, must be readily available to all members of the nursing staff on the patient care units. Only when they are understood and used can they be documented and audited.

Standards are intended to provide a basis for measurement which is objective, achievable, practical, flexible and acceptable. One type of standard is broad in nature and serves a particular kind of purpose in providing guidelines. These are structure standards, such as those provided by ANA and JCAH.

Another and more specific type of standard or criterion is needed for the retrospective nursing audit. It identifies what element of care is being evaluated by an inspection of a patient's chart. An element of care that is of major consequence to the patient includes the expectation of this element's presence in a chart (i.e., yes or no; or 100% for always, and 0% for never). Exceptions must be clearly defined, as acceptable within the range of normal professional expectations.

THE NURSING AUDIT TECHNIQUE

Retrospective audit, as defined, attempts to determine the degree to which the patient's chart accurately reflects the quality level of nursing care received by the patient and whether or not the level of care given is clinically sound and meets a standard of optimal care achievable by the healthcare agency. The retrospective audit procedure may focus on either an outcome audit or a process audit—or both. The outcome audit identifies patient outcomes that are satisfactory or unsatisfactory and is intended to identify also the patterns of nursing care that appear to be responsible. The process audit is a deeper probe of already recognized or suspected problems in the nursing care process.

Outcome audits use as the elements for consideration two factors—Discharge Status and Complications. The three components of discharge status are health, activity and knowledge. In order to determine discharge status and complications, it is necessary to establish a base-line assessment. For this reason the audit committee may need to refer to the initial assessment (data base) to compare the patient's status at the time of discharge with his status at the time of admission.

A quantitative standard should be established for each component. The standard identifies the expected status of the patient in respect to each component at the time of discharge. The quantitative standard is always 100% for all assessment and discharge elements and 0% for complications. Exceptions, when stated, indicate the circumstances under which a condition that varies from the standard is justified.

The audit steps are:

1. The first step in the audit procedure is to establish standards and criteria. Standards are designed to provide measurement criteria and must be objective, achievable, practical, flexible and acceptable.
2. The second basic step is measurement. This means to secure the charts from Medical Records (possibly by random selection), excerpt the necessary data from the charts, then on a quantifiable basis demonstrate how well—by actual measurement—the results conform to the established criteria. This can be done by trained clerks once the procedure is established.
3. The third basic step is to evaluate the observable variations and decide which are justifiable in terms of the criteria and acceptable nursing practice and which are unjustifiable and represent actual deficiencies. Probable reasons for such deficiencies need to be established. This must be done by nurses.
4. Step 4 is to follow through with suitable corrective actions to prevent recurrence of such deficiencies. This is a most important part of the audit cycle, and one that is perhaps most difficult to handle. The efforts of a variety of personnel are required to carry out the action steps which may include direct one-to-one counseling, longer-range inservice education programs or modification of staffing in particular situations. In other cases the deficiency analysis may suggest clarification of or revisions in existing policies and procedures, or the development of new policies, forms or procedures.

5. Step 5 is the follow-through. This is the clincher, and answers the questions, "Did the action occur, and was it helpful in securing improvements?"
6. The sixth step, and the last of the six basic audit steps required by JCAH, is to prepare and distribute suitable summary reports to nursing service, hospital administration and to the executive committee of the medical staff.

As a management technique, then, nursing audit can be viewed as part of the evaluating and planning phases of the management process. It is ongoing rather than sporadic. Monthly and quarterly comparisons of results provide a way to determine the efficacy of the audit program.

AN APPLICATION IN PUBLIC HEALTH NURSING

Nursing audit is helpful in a variety of settings, not just in hospitals. The nurse manager in a public health agency needs to apply nursing audit as a facet of quality control. Applications in public health pose special kinds of challenges and opportunities. Public health nurses need to identify and set outcome standards for particular population groupings, such as the postpartum mother and infant, rather than for disease entities and surgical procedures. Another example of a particular population grouping is the high risk mother. Programs such as infant and child immunization and adult screening present another challenge and opportunity for the audit committee. Fortunately, nurses are developing innovative ways to meet the challenge while finding new job satisfaction in the process.

A pertinent example is the Cumberland County Health Department in Fayetteville, North Carolina. (Exhibits can be found in Appendix H.) The nursing director designated a nursing audit committee comprised of nine nursing staff members who had participated in a nursing audit workshop. Together they surveyed the literature, explored a variety of resources, and with the encouragement of their director used their ingenuity to initiate the audit program. The committee established the following goals and plan of action:

Short Range: Improve documentation of Maternal/Child Health records (initiated by MCH Program nurses) through setting nursing standards for MCH Records.
Long Range: Improve documentation of public health records through the establishment of nursing standards for all areas of

public health nursing and, through improved documentation, show proof of the quality of nursing care being delivered.

Steps to Achieving Goals:

1. Establish nursing standards for all areas of public health nursing.
2. Audit records for which standards have been established to determine quality of documentation.
3. Examine the results of the nursing audit and make recommendations regarding gaps in documentation (and possibly education) to supervisory personnel and nursing staff.
4. Execute follow- up and reassessment three to six months later.

Results of the public health agency retrospective audit and quality control check are shared with the maternal child health nurse based at the hospital and with the district public health nurses so that they can act on recommendations for improvement of the quality of care and the documentation of that care.

SECURING ACTION ON AUDIT REPORTS

One result of nursing audit analysis and problem identification is a recommendation for action to the person or department head who can make a decision and carry out the required implementation. Thus it is a committee responsibility to summarize a recommendation succinctly and to provide justification and support for the recommendation.

An effective tool to use for presenting recommendations is the Committee Follow-Through Memorandum (Exhibit 5:1). It requires reducing the recommendation to a relatively few words, and limiting the supporting justification to major items only, such as cost, benefits, suggestions for implementation. Thus for some recommendations that are rather extensive in their complexity and implications, the memorandum serves as a cover sheet for additional pages of audit findings, analysis results, estimates of cost and savings (if any), suggestions for methods of implementation and so on.

The principle that applies here is that of the doctrine of completed staff work. This means that the committee should be sure to do its homework. It should present the recommendation in such a way that the decision- making process becomes as easy as possible for the person to whom the memorandum is addressed. This can happen when the recommendation is simply and clearly stated and the justification is

Exhibit 5:1
Committee Follow-Through Memorandum

TO: ____ DATE: ______________

FROM: ____________________ , Chairman of ____________ Committee

SUBJECT: ____

Recommendation:

Justification *(Cost, benefits, suggestions for implementation)*:

(Attach supporting documents as necessary.)

- -

FOLLOW-THROUGH ACTION:

__________ Approved as recommended   ________ Disapproved for reasons as stated

__________ Approved with modification   ________ Referred back to committee

Comment:

Signed ________________________________   Date ______________

____

objective, incisive and persuasive.

In a very real sense the task of securing approval for a recommendation is a selling job. The following are guidelines for selling a desired course of action:

Make Ready: Know your prospect (needs, wants, goals).
Approach with Benefits: Answer the prospect's unspoken question, "What will this do for me?"
Stimulate Desire: Appeal to self-motivation. (Sell the sizzle, not the steak.)
Tell Facts: After the foregoing steps.
Eliminate Retardants: Forsee objections, remove them as obstacles.
Request Action: Ask for what you want done.

Then secure reactions and feedback, and follow through appropriately to assure action. Obviously the audit analysis and findings provide important facts, but they alone may not secure approval of the recommendations. So do your homework; complete your staff work by thinking through the implementation process that may be necessary; provide answers for the possible objections that may enter the decision-maker's mind (costs, complications, interdepartmental problems, legal or policy concerns, etc.) Make it as easy as possible to secure the answer you seek.

REPORTING AUDIT RESULTS

The sixth basic step in the audit procedure is to report the results of the auditing process periodically. This provides a record of the committee's work, a summary of audit activity, an organized presentation of general findings, the recommendations for action that have been presented, the follow-through action that has taken place and what has been the impact of such follow-through on the problem conditions.

One type of periodic report form is shown in Exhibit 5:2, the Audit Summary for a specific patient care unit. When this is used effectively by the nurse managers with personnel on the units through the Working Committees Plan, the audit program becomes a vital part of every employee's job. A main concern of most patient care personnel is the quality of care; and given the opportunity and leadership, they will contribute creatively to improving patient care practices.

The reporting function is a vital one in the auditing process. It provides a necessary communications link for feedback and evaluation purposes to the patient care units, nursing administration, hospital administration and the medical staff. Feedback of nursing audit results to the nursing staff on the patient care units is also essential. Audit committees must use a variety of methods for providing informative, useful feedback. An Audit Summary and the Committee Follow-Through Memorandum are written communications. Face-to-face verbal feedback is highly desirable too. Each audit committee member can become a personal ambassador to serve as a liaison between the committee and the head nurse or coordinator for one or more patient care units. Tactful, personal follow-through can add greatly to the effectiveness of the entire audit program.

A follow-up audit of the same audit topic should be carried out within a few months after recommendations and feedback have been given. The follow-up audit provides solid evidence of whether or not

Exhibit 5:2
Audit Summary

TO: Ward or Unit ________________________________ Date _________

FROM: Audit Committee   Signed _______________________ Chairman

RE: Audit Topic: ____

QUALITY CONTROL CHECK

________Number of Open Charts Audited

________Number of Patients Observed/Interviewed

________Number of Personnel Observed/Interviewed

RETROSPECTIVE AUDIT

________Number of Closed Charts Audited

FINDINGS AND RECOMMENDATIONS

1.   Indications of quality care:

2.   Outstanding problems:

3.   Indications of improvement:

4.   Recommendations for improvements:

5.   Special comments:

---

improved documentation and/or patient care quality has been achieved.

The feedback process is intended to be more than one-directional. The audit committee itself needs regular feedback and evaluation if it is to perform effectively and meet its responsibilities. When the committee seeks and encourages such feedback it is most likely to receive it. The evaluation of the audit committee's performance can be achieved through a variety of measures. These include a regular reporting of the quantity of audits performed, the quality of audits completed, a statistical comparison of findings and follow-through action and subjective evaluation of how well each of the stated committee purposes and objectives are being met.

NURSING AUDIT AND THE NURSE MANAGER

Auditing is an inspection process. It compares results withstandards and criteria. Thus it is a most useful tool for the nurse manager. Every organization requires its own relevant inspection procedures. In general manufacturing where the measurement of size and dimensions is critical, "go, no-go" gauges are used. The item is either satisfactory (within standard) or it isn't. In the auditing of patient care and patient records there is a similar identification of those elements of care which represent "go" or "no-go" quality. Elements are either to be present (100% STD) or not present (0% STD) for acceptable clinical performance. In a quality check of nursing care, a desired attribute is present or it isn't. Audit necessarily provides for acceptable variations for identifiable reasons. These too must be defined and documented as described earlier.

The guidelines for nursing audit take into account the variables among healthcare agencies and their relative performance capabilities. The thrust is for every agency to adapt to its own uses the fundamental philosophy and basic steps of nursing audit so that there can be demonstrable progress and improvements. Nurse managers welcome such programs for improving patient care through professional, business-like methods. Nurse managers make them work well for their intended purposes.

Nursing audit is only one part of the growing trend towards a system of nursing that has as its focus the prevention of illness and care of patients based upon their identified problems and needs. In such a problem-oriented system it is essential to establish outcome and process standards of care as a basis for nursing practice, nursing documentation of that practice and the auditing of both the practice and the documentation. The success of such a system rests largely upon the ability of nurse managers to assure that nurses utilize effectively the nursing process (assess, plan, implement, evaluate) on a continuous basis in all patient situations.

Goals and objectives need to be mutually set and agreed upon by nurses and patients (along with other health professionals) so that everyone is working toward the same ends. MBO and Nursing Management by Objectives blend well with the problem-oriented system and its audit component. After all, standards and objectives have much in common, even by definition. It is timely to begin involving the patient and his family more directly in establishing objectives. Nurses must plan and carry out patient care with the patient whenever possible, rather than at or for the patient.

Job satisfaction is essential for the nurse. Results-oriented performance evaluation, based on the philosophy and principles of MBO, adds another personally satisfying dimension and provides for feedback and self-evaluation of performance with patients. ROPEP rests solidly on the establishment of standards of personnel performance. Coupled with standards of nursing care for use on the patient care units and for nursing audit purposes, there is the promise of being able to maintain a consistently satisfactory level of quality in nursing staff performance and patient care. Nursing audit, as one means of measuring quality of care, is a healthy indicator for the future direction of nursing and patient care under the leadership of professional nurse managers.

NOTE

1. Marion E. Nicholls. "Quality Control in Patient Care," *American Journal of Nursing*, 74 (March 1974), pp. 456-59.

SUGGESTED READINGS

Books

Brunner, L.S. and Suddarth, D.S. *The Lippincott Manual of Nursing Practice* (Philadelphia: J.B. Lippincott Co., 1974).

Carter, J.H.; Hilliard, M.; Castles, M.R.; Stoll, L.D.; and Cowan, A. *Standards of Nursing Care: A Guide for Evaluation*, 2nd ed., enlarged. (New York: Springer Publishing Co., 1976).

Easton, Richard. *Problem-Oriented Medical Record Concepts* (New York: Appleton-Century-Crofts, 1974).

Froebe, Doris, J. and Bain, R. Joyce. *Quality Assurance Programs and Controls in Nursing* (St. Louis: C.V. Mosby, 1976).

Ganong, Joan and Warren. *HELP with Nursing Audit* (Chapel Hill, N.C.: W.L. Ganong Co., 1975).

Health Law Center. *Nursing and the Law* (Germantown, Md.: Aspen Systems Corp., 1975).

Jacobs, Charles M. and Nancy D. *The PEP Primer* (Chicago: JCAH, 1975).

Mayers, Marlene. *A Systematic Approach to the Nursing Care Plan* (New York: Appleton-Century-Crofts, 1972).

Mayers, Marlene G. *Standard Nursing Care Plans* (Palo Alto, Calif.: R/P Co., Medical Systems, 1974, 1975).

Mazur, W.P., MD. *The Problem-Oriented System in the Psychiatric Hospital* (Garden Grove, Calif.: Trainex Press, 1974).

Neelon, R.A., MD and Ellis, G.J., MD. *A Syllabus of Problem-Oriented Patient Care* (Boston: Little, Brown & Co., 1974).

Nursing Clinics of North America. I. *The Problem-Oriented Record.* II. *Quality Assurance.* (Philadelphia: W.B. Saunders Co., 1974).

Phaneuf, M.C. *The Nursing Audit: Profile for Excellence* (New York: Appleton-Century-Crofts, 1972).

Vasey, Ellen and Riley, Mary. *Quality Assurance: Peer Review for Nursing* (Pittsburgh: Western Pennsylvania Regional Medical Program, 1975).

Woolley, F.R.; Warnick, M.W.; Kane, R.L., and Dyer, E.D. *Problem-Oriented Nursing* (New York: Springer Publishing Co., 1974).

Weed, L.L. *Medical Records, Medical Education, and Patient Care* (New York: Appleton-Century-Crofts, 1972).

Yura, H. and Walsh, M. *The Nursing Process* (Washington, D.C.: The Catholic University of America Press, 1967).

Article

Kerr, Avice H. "Nurses' Notes: That's Where the Goodies Are," *Nursing '75* (February 1975), pp. 34-41.

Chapter 6
Annual Budgetary Planning

BUDGETING AND THE MANAGEMENT PROCESS

Budgeting is planning; budgeting is doing and implementing; budgeting is controlling, measuring and evaluating. Budgeting is the essence of managing. The budgeting process not only embraces the three functions that comprise the management process; the budgeting process, to a large extent, influences and measures the degree of success with which managers carry out their managerial responsibilties. In the Chapter 8 presentation of the 5M Formula, you will see that the "Big M" is the nurse manager who has a multiplying effect upon the utilization of the three Ms of manpower, materials and machines. But the fifth M, money, pervades all elements of the formula, including the R for results. Money is the least common denominator of all that managers do. Money is the ultimate unit of measure. Budgeting has to do with the flow and utilization of money.

Cash flow refers to the rate at which monies are received and spent. Every household manager has experienced a cash flow problem when the rate of money coming in for a period of time has been less than the rate of spending for the same period of time. The problem is acute when no reserves are available to be drawn upon for that portion of current expenses not covered by current income. Hospitals experience the same difficulty. A front page story entitled "Providers Clamor for Stalled Medicaid Checks," in *The News and Observer*, a Raleigh, N.C. newspaper, for May 28, 1976 read in part, "Anxious nursing home and hospital administrators called Thursday for quick resolution of a Medicaid contract dispute that is tying up more than $3.3 million they are due for treating low-income patients.... Switchboards at the state office were swamped Thursday with calls from concerned hospitals and other healthcare providers—some complaining that they urgently needed their checks in order to meet their payrolls."

Nursing administrators and managers in the typical hospital have no capability or responsibility to influence the rate of income received by the hospital. The group that has the most significant influence upon the volume of hospital income and the rate at which it is received is the medical staff, since it is the doctors who provide the patients and who influence when the patients enter the hospital and how long they stay there. And it is the patients, whose hospitalization initiates the payment process, that provide (through whatever payment channel) the greatest portion of the hospital's income. But even though the doctors largely control the initiation of the income-producing process, they play little or no direct role in spending or controlling the operating expenses of the hospital—except insofar as they use the hospital facility and personnel in the pursuit of their hospital-related medical practice.

Operating expenses, the day-to-day costs of maintaining and running a hospital or other healthcare agency, are considered to be controlled by hospital administration and the department heads. In fact, it is the people who work in the hospital, all of the employees at every level, who spend the money that makes up the greatest portion of the operating expense budget. This is a stark and simple fact. The employees use up the minutes and hours of each working day that are translated into payroll dollars, the largest single item of operating expenses. And employees are the ones who spend the money that was paid for materials and supplies, since they are the people who actually use those supplies and materials in doing their daily work. Employees, therefore, individually and as an entire group, control a major portion of the expenditure of the hospital monies, because in the most literal and realistic sense they are the ones spending and using up the hours, supplies, materials and other components of operating costs. A payroll clerk or an accounts payable clerk may write the checks, but they have little or no control over the actual expenditure of the money.

All but the most unobservant managers recognize the truth in the statement, "Your people can pull the rug out from under you any time they want to." It's true. Your people can help you or prevent you from achieving your objectives. Your people can help you or prevent you from controlling your expense budget, because they control what happens to every dollar more than you do. This is what Douglas McGregor was saying in his hard-hitting article, "Do Management Control Systems Achieve Their Purpose?"[1] McGregor concluded that traditional management control systems often fail because of non-compliance by employees who perceive in such systems the threat of punishment, lack of trust and a negative impact on their own human needs. They retaliate simply by not complying with demands for change, using their own imagination to beat the system and sometimes fudging the data as part of the numbers game to distort the control reports.

McGregor's recommendations for a managerial strategy for inducing employee involvement and commitment are summarized in Chapter 3. The theme of this book and our reasons for including so much of the humanistically oriented philosophy, techniques and principles of managerial leadership are related directly to McGregor's message. These techniques and principles are directly related also to the findings of other realistic researchers, and to our own work experiences and observations of organizational behavior. Budgetary planning and control (in the sense of feedback, measurement and evaluation) provide the management technique which, fully utilized, serves as the bottom-line indicator of the caliber of managerial leadership and performance.

THE NURSE MANAGER'S ROLE IN COST CONTAINMENT

Nurse managers, given the information and tools to use, quickly learn to recognize the validity of this viewpoint and to discharge their budgetary responsibilities with expertise. This chapter is devoted to budgeting as related to operating expenses because this is the portion of the total budget over which nurse managers have major influence. They can do something about operating expenses. They have little or no control over the capital budget—the planned expenditures for major projects, items of equipment or facilities that will be amortized rather than being paid for as part or the current year's expenses. Yet nurse managers need to be sufficiently familiar with the budgeting procedure for capital items so that they can submit budgetary requests for equipment or facilities when they believe they can be justified on a cost/benefit basis or for their expected contribution to patient care programs. Thus the major part of this chapter is devoted to annual budgetary planning and control from the point of view of nurse managers who have—or should have— this responsibility for their own patient care units, sections or departments.

The significance of the nurse manager's fiscal responsibility is dramatized through a Financial Organization Chart for the nursing service operating expense budget in a department of nursing. The first example, Figure 6:1, is a university hospital of approximately 350 beds. The total annual operating budget of 5.7 million dollars, for which the director of nursing has responsibility, is approximately 40% of the

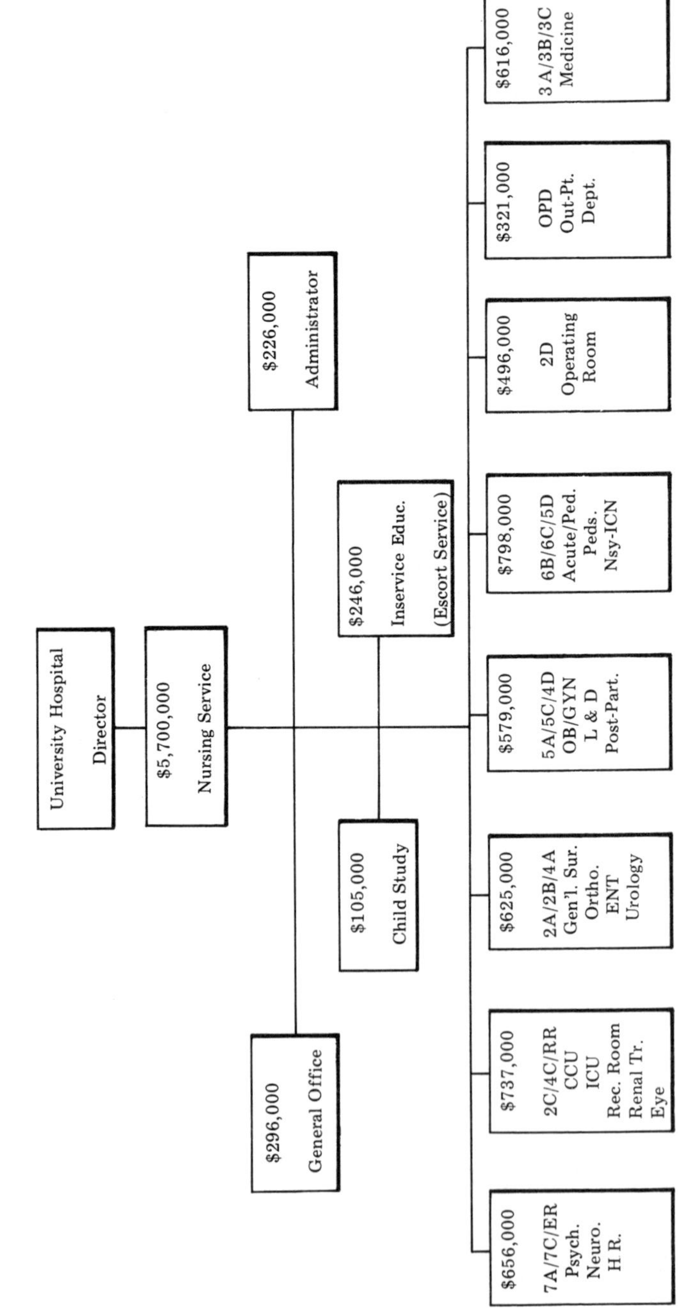

Figure 6:1

A Financial Organization Chart for Nursing Service Operating expense Budget, 1975-1976
(All figures to nearest thousand dollars.)

total operating budget for the entire hospital—a percentage quite typical for general hospitals in the 300- to 500-bed size category. Variations of a few percent from this figure are usually due to the inclusion or exclusion of certain departments (OR or Central Supply, for example) in the nursing service budget.

Note in the example that the patient care units are grouped in eight clusters, each group having its own nurse manager reporting to the director of nursing. These eight nurse managers have individual responsibility for operating budgets ranging from $321,000 to $798,000, depending upon the number, size and nature of the patient services offered in each group of units. Payroll expenses alone make up over 90% of the operating expenses for this department of nursing. Here again, the percentage is typical for comparable hospitals. No wonder, then, that escalating wages over the past decade have had such an impact on the costs of hospitalization. And no wonder that nurse managers have been exhorted to operate with the minimum size of staff, use the lowest salary classification of personnel who can do the work, avoid scheduling staff for overtime work and take advantage of every other means possible to contain payroll expenses. Many nurse managers feel with considerable justification that they have been fighting a losing battle because of the wage/price spiral, the state of the economy, and the difficulty (in many areas) of recruiting the kind and quantity of personnel to build stable, competent patient care teams.

In the second organization chart example, Figure 6:2, the arrangement of the unit clusters and the reporting relationships as shown were developed by the nurse managers to meet existing needs and opportunities and to serve as the basis for a longer-range developmental plan. The chart indicates that responsibility for day-to-day operations is shared by two associate directors reporting to the director of nursing service. The head nurses report either to a supervisor or directly to one of the two associate directors. The clinical specialists also report to one of the two associate directors and serve in a staff capacity for their respective unit clusters. As clinical specialists, they are available also to the entire department when their individual clinical skills are required. The projected operating expenses for the fiscal year have been added to the chart. The recommendation and rationale for adopting the organizational plan as shown was as follows:
Recommendation: Adopt the organizational structure depicted on the attached chart effective July 1.

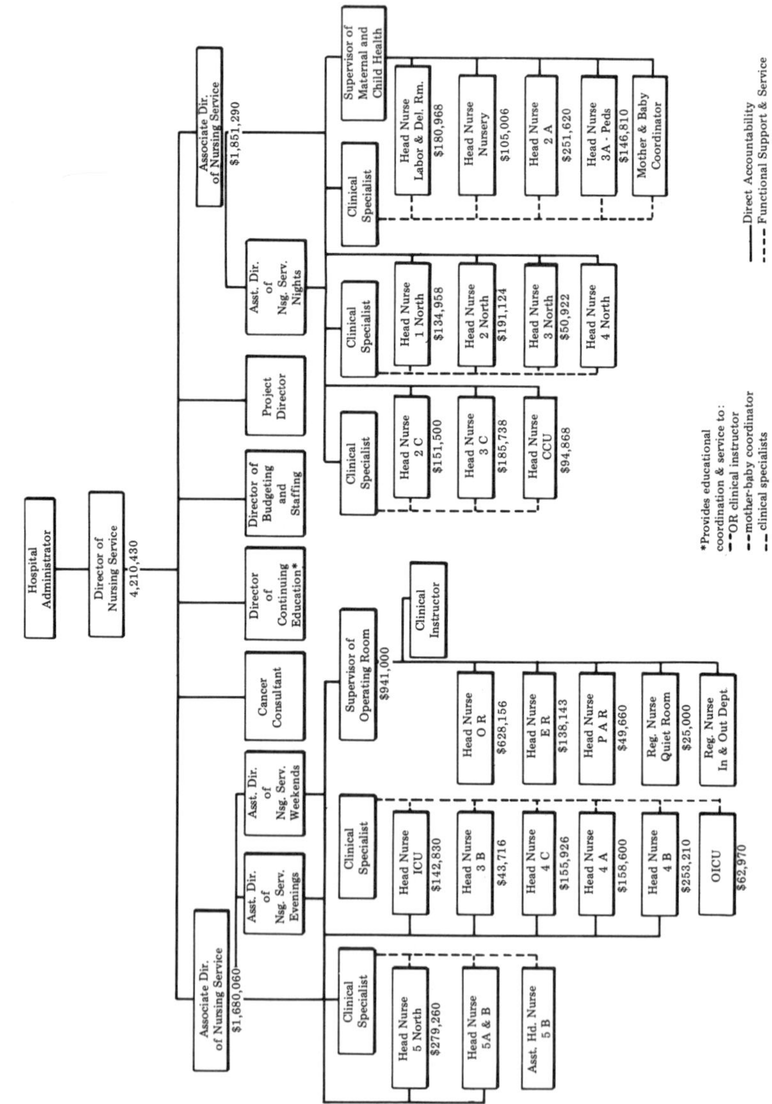

Figure 6.2
Budgetary Control Responsibility within the Department of Nursing

Rationale: This organizational plan—
1. Provides maximum capability to support cost containment goals of administration;
2. Continues our hospital's tradition of providing the best in patient care;
3. Builds upon the assets and demonstrated potential of nursing personnel;
4. Provides for flexibility and rapid response to changing demands and conditions;
5. Has the built-in mechanism for effective budgetary control;
6.Vests authority and accountability in those key nursing personnel who have responsibility for day-to-day operations and patient care;
7. Provides adequate and competent staff support to the nurse managers; and
8. Strengthens the department's ability to achieve interdepartmental, hospital-wide communications and cooperation.

Chapter 7, in the section on organizing for motivational management, presents additional concepts and considerations relating to organizational structure. Budgeting and cost containment will continue to be vital areas of concern for nurse managers. To cope with these matters, nurse managers deserve the best practical staff support and service that can be made available. Some nursing departments are providing such help within the department of nursing by establishing a position of Coordinator of Systems and Planning, or comparable title. A performance description is included in Appendix G. Persons in such a position, suitably qualified, earn their salaries many times over each year through savings and improvements in staffing, methods and procedures, work simplification, new product analysis and so on. They are nursing management engineers, with or without portfolio. They provide vital supporting services on demand to the nurse managers who have the direct fiscal responsibility on each unit, unit cluster, section and division of the nursing department. Working together, they can demonstrate laudable results in operational management.

Nurse managers can set up simple graphs and charts (e.g., man hours/patient day, operating expenses/month) to help control expenses on a day-to-day basis and contribute to real cost containment results. In our experience an organizational approach works better than a more limited systems, technically-oriented approach. The organizational approach is one which places responsibility for fiscal management in the nurse managers at every level and provides them with what they need to carry out that responsibility. Under such circumstances the nurse manager delivers often unforeseen, commendable results in money management and patient care.

In a larger context, nurse managers need to understand and cooperate with broad-scale cost containment efforts such as those described by Theodore Levitt in his article "The Industrialization of Service." Levitt explains how a sufficient total volume of activity permits applying the "principle of magnitude"; then systems and techniques can be used which produce reliable, rapid, and low unit-cost service results. He cites some specific healthcare examples.

1. Specialized, highly automated medical diagnostic clinics. The Damon Corporation in Needham Heights, Massachusetts, operates 125 such clinics throughout the nation in which, with the help of modern machines, 125 salaried M.D.s, 22 Ph.D.s and 1,400 medical technologists perform a wide range of diagnostic tests that formerly required patients to visit several doctors and clinics at costs in time and money several multiples above those of Damon's.

2. Prepaid health service centers, consisting of a wide range of specialists who can be kept fully employed at their specialties. Pioneered by the Kaiser Foundation in Oakland, California, there are several hundred Health Maintenance Organizations all over the country. Members prepay annual "dues" for easy access to full-time medical specialists and technicians working in central clinics (equipped with the latest technology) at their respective specialties, and only their specialties. Nor is the low-cost, rapid, convenient health care confined to outpatient services. Since the formation of a first Ambulatory Surgical Facility in Phoenix, Arizona in 1970, there are now nearly 100 ASFs in the United States. These are normally equipped to do some 125 low-risk operations on patients. The typical facility has two or more operating rooms, a recovery area, and a diagnostic center. The patient comes in (say for a tonsillectomy), undergoes tests and surgery, rests, and goes home — all in one day.

For example, at Northwest Surgicare, a for-profit ASF in the Chicago area, the total tonsillectomy bill is $169 compared with $548 at Chicago's not-for-profit Michael Reese Hospital. The Metropolitan Insurance Company, which honors 22 ASFs under group insurance policies, estimates it has saved $1 million in the past three years.[3]

The remainder of this chapter is devoted to an organized approach to which every nurse manager can contribute—annual budgetary planning and control on a year-round schedule as part of each one's responsibilities for patient care programs and human resources management.

INTRODUCTION TO ANNUAL BUDGETARY PLANNING (ABP)

When we first wrote about "ABP for Nursing Administration,"[2] we used ABP as the abbreviation for Annual Business Plan, a deliberate carry-over of a term used in general business situations for the type of comprehensive planning process described. Our reason for using "business" in the title was twofold: (1) in an industry (healthcare) usually cited as the first or second largest in the country the time is long overdue for coming to grips with the business issues involved, using the appropriate terminology for doing so; and (2) nurse managers recognize that the business of healthcare organizations is patient care and that businesslike plans of care and businesslike methods for the delivery of such care lead to best results for patients and consumers generally.* We find no one to dispute that position with any serious conviction.

The pace of change being what it is, however, we take no umbrage with those nurse managers who are not yet ready to adopt the Annual Business Plan terminology for use within their own nursing department. This is in recognition of the fact that even today in far too many hospitals the nurse managers play little or no significant role in budgetary planning and control. In such hospitals the use of an ABP program for annual budgetary planning with realistic involvement of the nurse managers is a major progressive step toward improved hospital-wide management.

In other hospitals we find situations in which an administrator, controller or business manager is far too ready to pass over to the nursing administrator a disproportionate share of the burden for budgetary matters. In view of the fact, therefore, that annual business planning is necessarily a hospital-wide function, this chapter presents ABP in that context, but with the focus on the nurse manager's role in budgetary planning and control. As stated in the first sentences of AHA's 1961 publication *Budgeting Procedures for Hospitals*, "Planning future operations through budgeting is an integral part of suc-

---

* For a scholarly, documented analysis supporting this view, see "The Industrialization of Service" in the *Harvard Business Review*, 54 (Sept.-Oct. 1976), pp. 69-70.

cessful businesses today. Similar planning is equally important to successful operation of our hospitals."[4]

Figure 6:3

Annual Budget Plan (ABP) For Department of Nursing*

Fiscal Year July 1, 1977-June 30, 1978

SCHEDULE / ACTIVITIES	JUL	AUG	SEP	OCT	NOV	DEC	JAN	FEB	MAR	APR	MAY	JUN	WHO WILL DO/HELP
1. Establish Objectives for the Fiscal Year 1977-1978	■												Dir. of Nursing Assoc. Director
2. Identify Key Issues	■	■											Dir. of Nursing Assoc. Director Pt. Care Coords.
3. Analyze Performance and Resources		■	■										Dir. of Nursing Controller Pt. Care Coords.
4. State Basic Assumptions			■	■									Pt. Care Coords. Dir. of Nursing
5. Set Unit Objectives					■								Pt. Care Coords. Unit Staff
6. Develop Program Strategies and Action Plans						■	■						Pt. Care Coords. Unit Staff
7. Forecast Income						■	■						Controller
8. Develop Operational Plans								■	■				Pt. Care Coords. Unit Staff
9. Prepare Budget Recommendations									■				Pt. Care Coords. Dir. of Nursing Assoc. Director
10. Submit Budget; Review, Revise, and Secure Approval										■	■		Dir. of Nursing Assoc. Director Pt. Care Coords.

*Adapted from Joan and Warren Ganong, "ABP for Nursing Administration," *Journal of Nursing Administration*, 3 (May-June 1973), p. 6.

Figure 6:3 presents a program performance plan for a nursing department's annual budgetary plan considered as part of the hospital's annual business plan.   The time span shown is the twelve-month period preceding the beginning of a new fiscal year on July 1. The July through June fiscal year is the one most commonly used in hospitals. The sequence of steps in the ABP process is listed from top to bottom in the Activities column while the scheduled time for carrying out each step is shown by the horizontal block spanning the projected number of weeks required. The titles in the "Who will do or help" column indicate the persons who will assume primary responsibility for completing the particular planning activity by the scheduled date. Specific titles for a given hospital will vary with the size and nature of the agency. For example, a nurse with the title of Coordinator for Systems and Planning, reporting to the director, can become a key person in the ABP process. This title would be substituted for associate director and/or others when such a person is part of the staff. The director of nursing has responsibility for maintaining the schedule whether the persons with the titles indicated are members of the nursing department or not. Missed due dates will seriously impair the orderly progression of the entire planning sequence. The numbered paragraphs that follow relate to the numbered activities in Figure 6:3.

1.Establish the departmental objectives for the fiscal year. For every year these objectives stem from the goals of the nursing department. The objectives for each year are stated as the specific operational results which the nursing department intends to accomplish, and are related to the long-range planning for the entire hospital as enunciated by the administrator or other chief operating executive. Such objectives are more quantitative and measurable than those usually included in the typical statement of philosophy and objectives which a nursing department has in its existing manuals. When a management-by-objectives program is in effect, the annual objectives are part of the MBO plan. Such objectives are the stepping stones of progress leading to the achievement of the broad departmental goals for the fiscal year.

Example: One nursing objective is to select a patient care coordinator for each of two pilot groupings of related units (maternal and child care, and three medical-surgical units) as a step toward better utilization of all personnel while maintaining or improving the quality of patient care. The related hospital objective, part of the administrator's annual business plan, is to move toward more decentralized management of hospital departments having similar operational characteristics and problems for the purpose of cost containment and more effective performance.

2. Identify key issues. Key issues are factors that need identification because of their likely impact upon the operation of the patient care units during the year. The following key issues have obvious implications for the entire hospital business plan for the year.

Examples: (A.) The planned retirement of a well-liked neurosurgeon with a large practice, with no replacement in sight, will affect the OR schedule and the surgical floor census.

(B.) The imminent merger of this hospital with another will affect the nursing department's organizational relationships; formal completion of incorporation is expected early next year.

(C.) Organizing attempts by two different labor unions that seek to represent nurses will likely result in an election before the end of this year.

3. Analyze past performance, available resources, expected demands, and known constraints. This involves three major aspects. The first is the review of past performance results, existing organizational assets and resources, and a realistic assessment of limitations and constraints affecting the scope of realistically obtainable objectives. This first step is an inward look at your own organization. It is a kind of intra-organizational audit.

Example: Assume an objective of adding four beds to an existing 10-bed ICU, to be effected by August 1. In order to estimate the effect of the four additional beds on the operating expenses per bed, an examination must be made of current operating expenses per bed in the existing 10-bed ICU as related to occupancy rate, trend of supply costs, and physician attitudes toward the use of the unit for their patients. The 40% increase in bed capacity may result in an increase of operating expenses per bed by an amount significantly less than or greater than the 40% increase in the number of beds. The accuracy of the forecast and its influence on the nursing budget depend largely upon how well this analysis is carried out.

The second aspect is an outward-looking step. It is a type of community-oriented survey to update your knowledge of your market, to use a respectable business term. It answers such questions as: Who are your consumers of patient care? What are their characteristics — age, sex, culture, socioeconomic status, health status, etc.? What services have they been using in what volume? What community changes may affect the mix of such services that should be available in the year ahead?

> *Example:* A large influx of younger families into new real estate developments in the hospital area is causing an increasing use of the OB, GYN, PEDS, and ER departments. This will influence space, equipment, and staffing requirements for the year ahead.

The third aspect is competition analysis, also an outward-looking step. It provides information about other healthcare agencies in your market area and what their plans are so that your hospital and nursing department can intelligently relate such information to your own planning.

> *Example:* The recent opening of a private nursing home in your area last summer is expected to reduce the pressures to expand your extended care facility. The new nursing home, together with the plans of other community agencies and the opening of a retirement village in another town, may dictate maintaining the present size of your own extended care facility or even a planned reduction in such service.

4. *State Basic Assumptions.* These are expectations which must be stated in writing, to avoid embarrassing and costly misunderstandings, communication breakdowns and failure to attain an objective. The basic assumptions in this plan should be prepared by the end of November by each patient care coordinator.

> *Examples:* (A.) Mrs. Acey will be available to become the patient care coordinator of units 7, 8, and 10 to replace the supervisor who is moving to Florida in the fall of this year.
> (B.) The supply of trained LPN's being supplied by local sources can be increased by fifteen per cent per month beginning September 1.
> (C.) Some form of mandatory rate control will be instituted in this state by the springtime two years from now.

5. *Set Unit Objectives.* The unit objectives are the specific operational results which each unit plans to accomplish during the fiscal

year. Such objectives reflect objectives of the department of nursing as set forth in Step No. 1, but are translated into detailed terms specific to each unit. These objectives are prepared by the patient care coordinator of each unit, to be completed no later than December 31.

Examples: (A.) Install additional autoclave in C.S.R. (Expected delivery date is early September.)
(B.) Prepare LPN's to assume an increasing share of technical duties. (Program plans and dates to be supplied by inservice director and head nurses.)
(C.) Provide inservice programs for RN's on the problem-oriented nursing system (September through March).
(D.) Revise current cyclical schedule to provide for every other weekend off (effective date October 1).
(E.) Establish nursing audit standards and criteria for eight additional disease entities.

6. *Develop Program Strategies and Action Plans.* This step considers the strategies and tactics to be used in each unit's "marketing" program (service offerings and how to interest potential users in them). The input of prior steps provides the necessary data for the formulation of the action plans and strategies. The unit profile (described in Chapter 7) can be helpful also. This step is necessarily a coordinated effort by the patient care coordinator of each unit, with the help of the director of nursing service and pertinent members of the medical staff working closely within the policies and objectives of the institution. The completion date is the end of February two years hence.

Example: The OB department will initiate a planned program beginning October next year to better compete with the "loss-leader" (services below cost) services of a local proprietary hospital that has affected the census in OB and related income. Possible activities include closer contacts by the admitting department with the appointment secretaries in the offices of OB/GYN physicians, a stepped-up teaching program for expectant mothers, and a follow-through service to involve the visiting nurse association together with an information program to publicize these services.

7. *Forecast Income.* The income forecast is an essential ingredient of the budgetary plan in order to predict: (a) how achievement of stated objectives may increase or decrease the amount of income for the year; (b) where the money is coming from to pay for the costs of approved programs related to specific objectives. The nursing department usually has little or no responsibility for direct input to this step. The income forecast is to be developed by the controller during January and February.

> *Example:* The planned program for OB services (see example in step 6 above) is expected to make little impact on the OB census during the coming fiscal year and will cost approximately $3,000. The expectation for the following year will be increased utilization and income of about 10%.

8. *Develop Operational Plans.* These plans set forth in as much detail as possible the full annual plan prepared by each unit to achieve the approved objectives. Completed by March 31st, this plan permits budget preparation in time for board approval prior to the beginning of the new fiscal year.

> *Example:* An operational plan includes a twelve-month timetable of activities, staffing requirements and schedules, recruitment efforts, utilization of agency resources, services required from other internal or external sources, rate of expenditure of funds and so on.

9. *Prepare Budget Recommendations.* The budget summarizes in dollars what the ABP means in terms of income and expenditures. It projects the rate of expenditure of funds allocated to permit progress toward established objectives and provides a measure of performance results on a monthly basis.

> *Example:* If none of the $3,000 allocated for the OB program (see examples in steps 6 and 7) has been spent by the February date, then performance progress on this objective will be behind schedule and require review and possible rescheduling.

10. *Submit Budget; Review, Revise, and Secure Approval.* This is the last step in the ABP process. In far too many hospitals, Steps 9 and 10 are considered to be the sum and substance of annual budgetary planning. Note that with ABP, the budget is simply the

outcome of the foregoing steps that provide the basis for the budget itself.

THE MEANING OF ABP FOR NURSE MANAGERS

It should now be clear why the term Annual Budget Plan is so meaningful for nurse managers as part of the hospital's annual business plan. ABP really refers to your annual management plan for the nursing department. The budgeting process, carried out as described by the ten-step program performance plan, brings together all of the elements of the nursing management process—the unifying theme throughout this book.

ABP is a technique which, like the other management techniques, helps nurse managers to carry out their management functions of plan, do and control. Each management technique provides particular help with one or more functions. And each technique in itself contains all three elements of planning, doing and controlling.

Here is a summary of how the ABP technique relates to, and involves a balanced use of, other nursing management techniques:

- Management by Objectives: ABP is the essence of MBO. Every objective has a price tag. The budget adds up the prices and helps decide upon the priority and scheduling of objectives.

- Problem-Oriented Nursing System: PONS has its focus on the patients and their care programs. The objectives for patient care programs are at the heart of all other hospital and nursing objectives, and become high-priority considerations in the ABP Steps 1 through 8.

- Results-Oriented Performance Evaluation Program: ROPEP is vital to Step 3 of ABP and to the nature and likelihood of achievement of the objectives, strategies, and operational plans developed in Steps 5, 6, and 8.

- Nursing Audit: Auditing is critical to the control aspects of MBO, PONS, ROPEP, and ABP.

- Motivational Management: Creating a motivational climate and a "motivating gap" (Chapter 7) are parts of a technique for nurse managers that influence especially the implementation and evaluation phases of ABP.

- Wide-Track Careers: The WTC program, as part of human resources management, is an ongoing part of every ABP. The success of WTC has a direct influence upon the nurse manager's success in using the other techniques too.

"Learning by doing," an age-old valid principle of education, has special meaning for those nurse managers who would learn budgeting. You will learn how to prepare and control budgets if you do it within your own agency, preferably with expert guidance. You may benefit from courses of instruction or from reading about the budgeting process if the content is specifically designed to meet your needs. In our experience, however, a far better investment of time is that spent in direct on-the-job training in preparing and controlling that portion of your agency budget for which you are responsible as a nurse manager. In so doing you will discover the true meanings and implications of all the other parts of this book dealing with your functions, techniques and skills as a nurse manager.

In summary, ABP as a year-round process brings together the techniques and functions of managing in a way seldom achieved previously so that nurse managers can comprehend, integrate, and carry out most successfully their responsibilities for patient care management, operational management and human resources management with professional confidence.

We can find no better way to conclude this chapter than to share the hard-headed, humanistic business philosophy expressed by Jimmy Carter in discussing zero-based budgeting during an interview with Norman Mailer. It explains a point of view and a method we believe urgently needs adoption in hospitals just as much as in government.

Mailer: I was fascinated with zero-based budgeting. It seems to me to make an awful lot of sense. As I understand it, a zero-based budget means that the head of any given bureau or department of government who has to prepare a budget cannot take anything for granted from previous years. Each year he has to reconstitute his budget, and list his priorities of need. So moribund little enclaves in his department tend to survive less. Is that correct?

Carter: That's correct. The only difference is that instead of beginning with a department head, it begins deep within the department, with a one-page form that's prepared by a shop foreman or a state patrol corporal or someone in charge of a seed laboratory. They analyze what they're doing and what their productivity ought to be, the output of their services, how many they hope to have the next two years. Same way with budget figures. Then there's a place for them to advocate improvements in the quality of their service or savings that would accrue from changes. It's a way for persons deep within a department, who've been there for 20 years and may not have ever met the department head, to say,

"This is what I think ought to be done..." It's a constant probing for a better way to do things, a constant assessment of priorities, and a constant winnowing out of the obsolescent or obsolete, or as you said, moribund programs. The other thing that we added on after the first year was an incentive reward program. People who made a proposal that saved the state money got 10 percent of the savings the first year. We put a maximum on it of a $2,000 reward. Periodically, I would have a little ceremony and present certificates of reward to those who did it. It makes the employees deep within the department, who've never in the past been involved, except to preserve the status quo—it makes them constantly probe for a way to do things better...

Carter:...You know, the thing that I was surprised to discover is that most of your civil servants are good people. Just like you and me. They've got one life to live and they've got one career to expend. I thought they would be my most adamant opponents when I began to put into effect zero-based budgeting. But I found they were my most avid supporters. They saw that for the first time in their lives in government service there would be a clear delineation of authority, a clear assignment of responsibility, a minimum of overlapping and duplication, a minimum of paperwork and red tape, and they could actually educate children and build highways or correct pollution problems or preserve their wild areas, you know, in a much more effective way. If they are highly professional, and most of them are, and they want to do a good job, they can say for the first time, "I have a right to recommend, without fear of retribution, some drastic changes or improvements in how I perform my own services." And this is a very good thing...beneath technique was invention, and the man at the bottom working at his job was not without invention. Creativity came from the roots and not the administration. The administration was there to cultivate the fields of possibility. It is the point of view that believes we search for justice because the passion for justice exists already within us, we are born with it. So it is also the point of view that creativity is not only in all of us but that we sicken and grow apathetic when we make no artful change in our environment.[5]

NOTES

1. Douglas McGregor, "Do Management Control Systems Achieve Their Purpose?" *AMA Management Review* (February 1967), p. 6.

2. Warren L. and Joan Mary Ganong, "ABP for Nursing Administration," *Journal of Nursing Administration,* 3 (May-June 1973), p. 6.
3. Theodore Levitt, "The Industrialization of Service," *Harvard Business Review,* 54 (Sept.-Oct. 1976), pp. 69-70.
4. E.N. Cappleman, *Budgeting Procedures for Hospitals* (Chicago: American Hospital Association, 1961), p. 1.
5. Norman Mailer, "The Search for Carter," *New York Times Magazine* (Sept. 26, 1976) pp. 83-85. Reprinted with permission.

SUGGESTED READINGS

Books

Cappleman, E.N. *Budgeting Procedures for Hospitals* (Chicago: American Hospital Association, 1971).
Cunningham, R.N. Jr. *Improving Work Methods in Small Hospitals* (Chicago: American Hospital Association, 1975).
Ganong, Joan and Warren. *HELP with Annual Budgetary Planning and Control* (Chapel Hill, N.C.: W.L. Ganong Co., 1976.).
Hospital Financial Management Association. *Planning the Hospital's Financial Operations: Readings in Hospital Budgeting* (Chicago: HFMA, 1972).
Hospital Financial Management Educational Foundation. *The Budgeting Process: Student Packet* (Chicago: HFMEF, 1970)
Marram, G.; Flynn, K.; Abaravich, W; and Carey, S. *Cost-Effectiveness of Primary & Team Nursing* (Wakefield, Mass.: Contemporary Publishing, 1976).
Sweeny, A. and Wisner, John. *Budgeting Basics* (American Management Association, 1975).
Trivedi, Vandenkumar M., *Hospital Management Systems Demonstration: Optimum Allocation of Float Nurses Using Head Nurses' Perceptions.* (Ann Arbor: Univ. of Michigan, Bureau of Hospital Administration, 1974).
Zollitsch, H.G. and Langsner, A. *Wage and Salary Administration* (Cincinnati, Ohio: South-Western Publishing Co., 1970).

Articles

Boer, Germain and Parris, Walter, "Flexible Budgeting—A Cost Control Tool," *Hospital Financial Management,* 24 (December 1970), pp. 12-14.

Boyarski, Robert P., "Nursing Workweek Equalizes Shifts, Time Off," *Hospital Progress*, 57 (July 1976), p. 36.

Ganong, Warren L. and Joan Mary, "ABP for Nursing Administration,"*Journal of Nursing Administration*, 3 (May-June 1973), p. 6.

Ganong, Warren L., Ganong, Joan M., and Harrison, Edwin T., "The 12-Hour Shift: Better Quality, Lower Cost," *Journal of Nursing Administration*, 6 (February 1976), p. 17.

Houser, Richard, "How to Build and Use Flexible Budgeting," *Hospital Financial Management*, 28 (August 1974), pp. 12-20.

Hospital Financial Management Association, "How to Build and Use a Flexible Budget," *Hospital Financial Management* (August 1974), pp. 12-20.

Journal of the American Hospital Association, "Greater Emphasis Placed on Sound Fiscal Management," *Hospitals*, 50 (March 1, 1976), p. 34.

Journal of the American Hospital Association, "Nursing Service Administrators: Times Call for Documentation," *Hospitals*, 50 (February 16, 1976), pp. 89-91.

Munch, Julia, "Let's Involve Nurses in Budget Planning!" *Hospitals*, 48 (February 16, 1974), pp. 75-78.

Part IV

Human Resources Management

Chapter 7
Motivational Management in Nursing

The nurse manager's responsibility for the management of human resources is involved with the self-development of oneself, staff and patients. It requires facilitating in the truest sense of the helping relationship. It includes providing growth opportunities for the givers and receivers of healthcare. It encompasses research, peer review, patient teaching, staff development and self-evaluation programs and learning projects. Human resources development is inherent in, and a major element of, two of the components of the problem-oriented nursing system — the foundation (principles of nursing practice) and education.

People who enter the healthcare arena for reasons of work or care bring with them all of their own values, needs, knowledge and skills. They come as workers to learn, to do, to help; or they come as patients for diagnosis, treatment, care, prevention of future health problems, and (when possible) to become involved in the planning, implementing and evaluating of their own care. The healthcare agency is a complex mixture of individuals with needs, problems, talents, feelings, faults, abilities, interests and life styles. Their motivations are of paramount interest in a discussion of human resources management.

THEORIES OF MOTIVATION

A theory is simply someone's idea about something, usually based upon a considerable amount of experience, study and research. Thus a theory of motivation attempts to provide a valid explanation of why people act the way they do. This is not the same as "causation" because motivation generally deals with a single class of events determining behavior. Causes may be many and varied. Motivation is different from ability, for example, which also influences behavior. You may be *able* to do something but not *want* to do it. Or you may *want* to do something but be *unable* to do it. For example, if while driving your car a crisis situation arises and you want to avoid an accident, you may be able to do so only if you can respond with the necessary mental and physical reflexes and skill. Thus both desire and ability combine to affect what you do. Undoubtedly you can name a variety of other factors that influence your behavior too. Motivation is ordinarily indicated by such words as want, wish, desire, need and striving.

The names of a number of researchers and scientists are identified with theories of motivation and human effectiveness. M. Scott Myers in *Every Employee a Manager* summarizes these theories by giving the name of the person identified with each theory, then grouping them in three categories. The first category includes those which focus on managerial styles and assumptions; the second describes combinations of managerial style and management systems; and the third describes the impact or consequences of styles and systems. In addition, the theories are presented on a low-to-high scale representing conditions ranging from those conducive to ineffective behavior at one end to conditions for greater effectiveness at the other.[1]

For example, Douglas McGregor's "Theory X" (reductive assumptions) is included as a managerial style having its impact at the ineffective end of the scale. "Theory Y" (developmental assumptions) is shown as leading to greater human effectiveness. Rensis Likert's "System 1" (exploitative authoritative) is in the same group at the ineffective end of the scale, with "System 4" (participative group) at the high effectiveness end of the scale.

Chris Argyris' "Autocratic Relationships" (conflict and conformity, alienation) is in the second grouping, and ineffective. "Authentic Relationships" (interpersonal and technical competence, commitment) is high effectiveness. Frederick Herzberg's concept of motivation-through-the-work-itself is in the second group too. "Environmental Comfort" (hygiene seeking) is ineffective; "Meaningful Work" (motivation seeking) is at the higher effectiveness end of the scale.

David McClelland's achievement motivation concept is in the third grouping. "Low Achievement" (more interest in things like affiliation, security, money, possessions) is less effective than "High Achievement" motivation (achievement is its own primary reward, high challenges, moderate risks, independence). Abraham Maslow's need hierarchy is also in the third group. "Lower-Need Fixation" (halted growth) is seen as providing lower human effectiveness than "Self-Actualization" (realizing potential).

Others included in Myers' summary are Blake, Hall, Bennis, Pare, Fromm and Glasser. The comparison is most useful since all of the theories have the common purpose of defining conditions which inhibit or enhance the expression of human talent. These theories, all of them carefully tested, can help nurse managers understand conditions for improved goal orientation and for the reduced—or more constructive—use of authority in achieving performance results.

All nurse managers need to have a personally comprehensible basis for their actions. They need to understand their own behavior. Just as important is the need to comprehend the behavior of others, to predict such behavior insofar as possible, and to make decisions and take actions that are most likely to produce the desired results in terms of goals and objectives. Your own education and experiences in living and working have provided you with some useful understandings about human nature and motivation. We suggest, however, that as a nurse manager you have a responsibility to yourself, your people and your agency to have a well-founded personal theory of motivation based upon your own experiences as well as upon the best research findings available to you.

We find that Maslow's durable theory of human needs as a basis for understanding human motivation works well for us. It rings true. It jibes with our experience. It is easy to use. It is positive in its impact. It provides an explanation for other motivational theories too. It gets good results for us. It can do the same for you. For these reasons, and because developing a sound working knowledge of Maslow's motivational ideas may be more useful to you than a smattering of knowledge about many theories, we focus on Maslow's work throughout this book. And we believe you will be able to adapt Maslow's theory to your own purposes. (See Appendix I.)

Motivation is a very personal matter. It stems from the needs of the individual. This is as true at work as it is in other areas of life. In a very real sense, then, you cannot motivate others; they motivate themselves. This helps to explain the frustration of so many managers, getting poor results in spite of their own dedicated efforts. "Why won't they do what I tell them? Why don't people care anymore? How can I ever get good work out of my people?"

Have you ever attempted to motivate another person only to discover that the other person (employee or patient) simply shows no evidence of being motivated? Have you asked yourself why your people seem not to respond; why they do not become motivated to do what you expect of them? Yet employees *are* motivated! They do act on the basis of what they feel as a desire, want, yearning, wish or lack. The problem, of course, is that too often their actions (insubordination, lack of interest, aggressive and unruly behavior, carelessness, quitting the job, joining the union) in response to what they feel as their needs, seem inimical to administrative goals and not in the best interests of patient care. What is the manager to do? How is the manager to satisfy organizational and patient-care goals while helping individuals at the same time to satisfy their own personal needs and goals?

THE NURSE MANAGER'S USE OF MOTIVATIONAL TECHNIQUES

A motivational technique is a way of encouraging actions that will assist others in meeting their needs while helping to achieve patient care objectives. The nurse manager who comprehends motivational technique has a potent force available for use. The technique involves identifying the currently felt needs of the other person, then helping that person to get what he wants—insofar as that is possible. Needs which are frequently unsatisfied—or poorly satisfied at best—include recognition, sense of achievement, enjoyment of the work itself, responsibility, advancement and growth. All of these are manifestations of the five Maslow-identified needs with which you are familiar.

Herzberg found that certain factors contribute to job satisfaction.[2] He called them the "motivators" or satisfiers. He found that other factors (organization policy and administration, supervision, work conditions, wages) contribute to job dissatisfaction. These he called the hygiene or maintenance factors. Note that an improvement in one or more of the maintenance factors may remove some causes for dissatisfaction but not contribute to job satisfaction! The opposite of job dissatisfaction in this case is not job satisfaction but no job satisfaction. Similarly, the opposite of job satisfaction is not job dissatisfaction but no job satisfaction. This distinction is significant in understanding Herzberg's findings and their impact upon motivational efforts by nurse managers and healthcare administrators.

He examined and summarized the factors affecting job attitudes reported in 12 investigations. He tallied those factors characterizing 1,844 events on the job that led to extreme dissatisfaction, as well as those factors characterizing 1,753 events on the job that led to extreme satisfaction. The major factors listed in rank order based upon their percentage frequency, are as follows:

Extreme Satisfaction	Extreme Dissatisfaction
1. Achievement	1. Company Policy and Administration
2. Recognition	2. Supervision
3. Work Itself	3. Relationship with Supervisor
4. Responsibility	4. Work Conditions
5. Advancement	5. Salary
6. Growth	6. Relationship with Peers

The motivational factors are not mutually exclusive. One builds on another. If employees express to you their need for advancement, you may find ways to allow them to grow and to recognize their achievement by recommending advancement. Then more than one motivator is being used. In each instance the individuals are being helped to meet their own human needs — and so they are self-motivated.

The use of such motivational factors can be a positive force in staying union free and in providing a better working climate in a unionized setting. The motivational factors must be understood and cultivated by the goal-oriented nurse manager. They may well become a part of your value structure and be built into your own goals and objectives for yourself at work. In addition, they deserve consideration when your agency, department or unit sets goals and objectives.

Because motivation is such a personal thing and people's needs vary from individual to individual, all people do not necessarily respond to the same appeals. Some people do not actively seek more responsibility or growth, for example. These same people may find satisfaction enough in the work itself. Such persons deserve continued encouragement; they may comprise a large segment of your workforce and meet their performance requirements satisfactorily.

The nurse managers, then, have to know their people. What works for one person at one time may not work for another person, or, indeed, for the same person at another time. Human needs shift in their priority. So you will need to be aware of such shifts and how they blend with the needs of your organization. People will be committed to your agency goals and objectives when they can identify how they tie in with their own needs. This is essential for the realistic application of motivational management concepts. Your use of motivational techniques must be genuine and open. The rewards can be felt in terms of job satisfaction for you and your people as well as better results in patient care and the delivery of patient care services.

If you agree with all of the foregoing, you may be wondering (as a pragmatic nurse manager) how to make it work for you. First of all, recall one of Maslow's early conclusions: "Success and reward have a far more powerful effect upon motivation than failure or punishment."[3] Secondly, follow the admonition of Peter Drucker, who said, "You cannot build on people's liabilities; you can build only on their assets."[4] Thirdly, identify and help people to satisfy their felt needs. When you comprehend, believe and act upon these three motivational precepts you can become a successful management motivator. You will be able to utilize the wisdom of Myers, who wrote, "People's behavior stems from their understanding of what they think they perceive."[5]

Recognize, too, that the model for motivational management technique, like the model for other management techniques, is built upon the three steps of the management process of plan, do and control.

The six motivational factors—achievement, recognition, work itself, responsibility, advancement, and growth—are those most frequently mentioned in the investigations summarized by Herzberg as characterizing job events that led to extreme satisfaction. The human needs are implicit in these factors. All three steps of plan/do/control in the motivational management cycle are action steps for the nurse manager: the nurse manager plans (mutually with the affected individuals) what specific needs, assets and opportunities exist now and in the immediate future for specific members of the nursing staff; the nurse manager interacts with the specific individuals, using the developed plan and related knowledge, and applies the three precepts cited above; the nurse manager gets feedback, measures results against expectations and follows through (all with direct involvement of the affected staff members). The cycle continues for these and other staff members. As with other techniques, once the pattern is established and practiced it becomes semi-automatic and spontaneous. But as with other techniques, the learning and initial implementation phases require special attention and extra effort.

For example, one way to practice the motivational management technique is to set up for each of your people (by name, dated) a sheet on which you simply list the motivational factors (and perhaps a specific, current, unsatisfied need) together with your thoughts of how specific motivators can be used and then your follow-through record. Such a sheet would include such items as these:

1. Achievement (successful accomplishment). Provide a work assignment (named) more consistent with demonstrated capabilities (named assets), challenging but with minimum risk of failure.

2. Recognition (acknowledgement, be aware of, sense of self-worth). Commend regularly for performance results. "You did a fine job of that (by name)." "That was really a great effort." "Good job." "Well done." "I appreciate your help. It means a lot to me." "You are really good at that." "What I like about you is...."

3. The Work Itself (intrinsic interest in and satisfaction with job content.) Improve job content to include more planning, self-direction and evaluation by (action). Coach the employee.

4. Responsibility (to be answerable for, accountability, sense of trust). Delegate responsibility and authority suitable to the individual (taking some calculated risks, allowing more freedom of action). Get feedback; be available, helpful, supportive as invited.

5. Advancement (to make progress; move forward; rise in rank, amount, value). Recheck person's own desires. Provide opportunities for special projects, new assignments as appropriate. Encourage person to qualify self for career-ladder opportunities. Use job enrichment concept in present job assignment. (Seek help from informed management engineer, systems analyst, or psychologist.)

6. Growth (to develop; become more capable). Provide fair opportunities to attend inservice, continuing education, workshops and related programs. Encourage further formal education and other learning opportunities based upon person's needs and expressed desires. Find ways to be able to say yes to requests. Seek assistance from inservice and staff development staff for on-the-job training designed for your own unit.

7. Social Need (affection, sense of belonging). An example might be a current unmet need because of recent separation and divorce. Give extra quota of special attention, as acceptable by person, during succeeding weeks and months. Possibly arrange invitation to home. Discuss options with personnel director or other interested persons.

ORGANIZING FOR MOTIVATIONAL MANAGEMENT

Healthcare organizations are living, dynamic, changing entities. They may be cumbersome, slow moving, and traditional; or innovative, quick to respond and attuned to environmental impact. While these words are used to describe organizations, they more accurately portray the agency director, administrator and other leaders who more than anyone else influence and project the image of the healthcare agency (and its major departments).

Maslow has said that he thought of creative management and creative education as developing the individual not only in terms of his own identity — his self — but also as part of his community, team, group and organization. In his writing on eupsychian management (i.e., human-oriented management enhancing psychological health), Maslow set forth thirty-six assumptions as preconditions to McGregor's theory of participative management.[6] The first of these is the assumption that everyone is to be trusted. Other assumptions are that people are not fixated at the safety need level, that people are improvable, that people prefer working to being idle, that all human beings prefer meaningful work to meaningless work. These assumptions, and the remainder of the list of 36, provide a provocative philosophical base for nurse managers in their discharge of their human resources management responsibilities.

It is obvious that some agency leaders will be more receptive than others to the management principles, concepts and techniques presented herein. The attitudes and values of the chief executive influence also the organizational structure itself and whether or not the structure contributes to or hinders goal achievement. These views are supported and emphasized by John F. Mee, who points out that effective performance of a manager requires a way of thinking, not the occupancy of a position.[7] Flexibility in adapting to change is essential in response to the changing economic, political, technological, social and ecological environments. But the ability of managers to respond to change and to assist other members of their management team to adapt to changing concepts of management is heavily influenced by: (1) the values and philosophy of the managers, especially as these affect behavior and decision making; (2) the kinds of knowledge and information possessed by managers; and (3) the abilities, skills and proficiencies possessed by managers. In fact, Mee asserts that managers of the future are likely to be evaluated more on the basis·of their value systems than on their knowledge and proficiencies.

Managers more and more are being considered as resource persons for those striving to achieve results, rather than being looked upon as authoritarian decision makers operating from the apex of a system of authority (as shown in a typical organization chart) who put their emphasis on an activities-oriented approach. By contrast, goal-oriented managers help to focus the achievement motivations of people toward accomplishing common objectives and realizing personal need satisfactions. The model Mee offers for a suitable organizational structure is shown in Figure 7:1.

Kraegel et al. supply a pertinent definition of organization as part of an introductory chapter to *Patient Care Systems:* "An *organization* is

Figure 7:1
Decentralized Results-Oriented Management

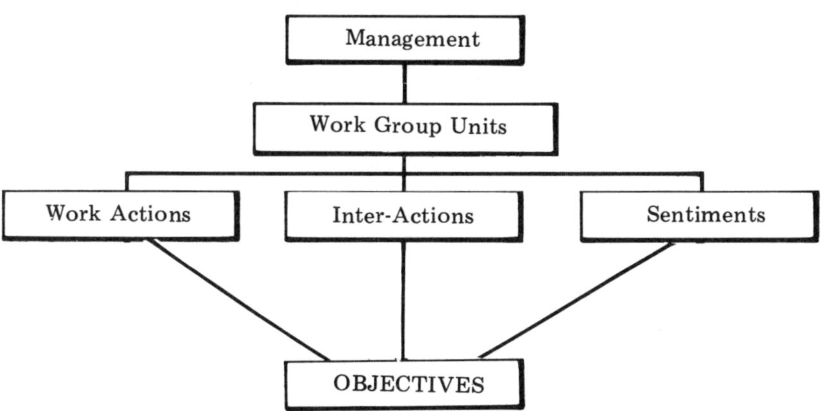

Adapted from John F. Mee, "Changing Concepts of Management, *S.A.M. Advanced Management Journal*, 37, no. 4 (October 1974), 22-34. Reprinted with permission.

defined as a system of interrelated resources, including environment, materials, supplies, and behaviors of people, that performs a task which has been differentiated into several distinct subsystems, each subsystem performing a part of the task, and the efforts of each being *integrated* to achieve effective performance of the total system."[8] The complexities of a hospital's interdepartmental and systems relationships dictate specific, purposeful action by top-level administration to establish the kind of dynamic integration that leads to unity of effort toward achieving the primary common purpose of meeting patients' needs. The problem-oriented nursing system is one of the vital systems contributing to the integrative plan.

When a nursing department decides to implement PONS, it is timely to carry out an objective review of the department's organizational plan and assignment of functional responsibilities. Some structures are better designed than others to provide the required support for a broadly based system such as PONS. What is usually called for is reorganizing the present structure, since the opportunity rarely exists to establish a new organizational structure from scratch. One of the dictums in architectural design is "Form follows function." The same principle applies in designing or redesigning the organizational plan of a hospital or a department of nursing: the plan of organization should fit the purpose of the organization and facilitate people's working together to achieve their goals and objectives. Problems and inefficiencies develop when an organizational structure, once adequate for an earlier time and environment, is no longer appropriate for today's demands. A "Model T" organization has no place on today's superhighway of modern healthcare. Yet some hospitals persist in attempting to adapt already outmoded organizational and systems models from general business or manufacturing industry in the name of modernization and progress. Results of such misguided attempts, predictably, often are more disastrous than they were when first developed for their original applications a quarter or half century ago.

As a nurse manager, consider the variety of factors having an impact upon departments of nursing as they influence organizational structure and performance. Such factors include:

1. Increasing demands and expectations from other professional groups and departments, ranging from hospital administration and the physicians to the younger generation of employees and labor unions.
2. The new period of stress and transition in the nursing profession itself as leaders strive to influence legislation affecting licensure; reduce intergroup dichotomy and fractionalization within the profession; and consolidate several sources of power so that nursing speaks with a stronger, more unified voice.
3. Greater clinical demands due to continuing increase in the technologies affecting patient care.
4. Burgeoning requirements of governmental, accrediting, educational, institutional, insuring and related agencies.
5. Critical necessity for cost containment through operational effectiveness in all areas.
6. The erosion of nursing's role in the delivery and management of patient care.
7. The pronounced thrust toward prevention rather than cure per se as the future emphasis in healthcare.
8. The human rights movement—here to stay in all of its manifestations—consumers, patients, employees, students, union members, managers, educators, doctors, nurses and all the other interrelated groups of which people are members.

These eight factors are discussed in other chapters. In total, they represent a substantial set of challenges to nurse managers. Traditional departments of nursing—structured with responsibility, authority and accountability highly centralized in the director's position—are not well positioned for coping with these challenges. Such an organizational structure, tending to rigidity and morbidity, is antithetical to the requirements for responding successfully to the ever-changing aspects of the aforementioned demands, challenges, trends, and opportunities.

What are the characteristics of an effective organizational structure for a nursing department that recognizes and wants to take appropriate initiative in acting upon the eight factors cited? Our suggestions are based upon assisting large numbers of nursing administrators and managers to move their nursing departments toward a more viable plan of organization. We believe an effective organizational structure for nursing meets the following criteria:

1. The organizational design has its focus on aiding the implementation of diverse, individualized patient care programs using the problem-oriented nursing system.

2. The structure is adaptive rather than monolithic; each unit or unit cluster may have its own unique way of organizing to meet its patient and personnel needs. For example, key functions (such as patient care programs, staffing, cost control) may be handled by the unit clusters rather than being fully centralized in the nursing office or fully decentralized to individual units.

3. True decision-making authority is held by nursing personnel at every level, especially by those closest to the patients.

4. Responsibility is not considered as delegated downward, but as an inherent component of each person's self-worth.

5. Accountability is first to oneself; all other aspects of accountability to others stem from this concept.

6. Problem solving is facilitated horizontally and vertically throughout the organization—the matrix model.

7. Power and communication centers are varied and dispersed—the homeostatic biological model.

8. The structure demands the use of motive force and innovative action from the greatest possible number of persons.

9. Systems changes are easily accommodated.

10. Interdepartmental communication and collaboration occur at all levels.

11. Intradepartmental coordination and control require minimal attention, but are effective through use of the management process at all levels.

12. Widespread nurse manager involvement in utilizing the management functions and techniques at all levels permits meeting current objectives while identifying and planning future goals for all three responsibilities of patient care management, operational management and human resources management.

No single structural concept will meet the requirements in all healthcare agencies. In one situation, for example, the department of nursing in a large state mental hospital redesigned their own organization and met most of the stated criteria. These nurses accomplished their goal by eliminating the position title of director of nursing and substituting a nursing committee elected by the RN's with cochairpersons. For a period of several years this committee form of elected leadership has met the needs of the nurses for more involvement in directing their own affairs, improving communications, and in solving their own problems.

Figure 7:2 shows a decentralized schematic organization plan evolved by the nursing department within a university medical center hospital. In this situation there was a recognized need for strengthening the posture and performance of the nursing department at all levels, while securing the benefits of productive dialogue, counsel and guidance from other professional university departments—notably the college of medicine, the medical staff, and the college of nursing. The diagram is an adaptation of the matrix model and provides the benefits of clearly defined channels of accountability within nursing (the solid vertical lines) and the necessary input and cooperation of the other professional departments (represented by the horizontal dash lines). The concept portrayed by the chart is important at all organizational levels, but especially so at the patient care unit level—which is "where the action is." Such a plan works most successfully when its purpose is understood; when the doctors, nurses, and educators want to make it work; and when the head nurses are strong, competent nurse managers who are skilled in all three areas of clinical, operational, and human resources management. When such conditions exist, there is the best possible environment to encourage nurse managers to become "excellent hospital integrators," as suggested by Marvin Weisbord.[9]

Any change in departmental structuring involves the redefinition of position responsibilities. Even a single change in the structure has multiple ripple effects upon the interrelationships of many persons and groups. When the change embraces moving from an authority-oriented centralized structure to one that is goal-oriented and

Figure 7:2
University Hospital Department of Nursing
Decentralized Schematic Organization Plan

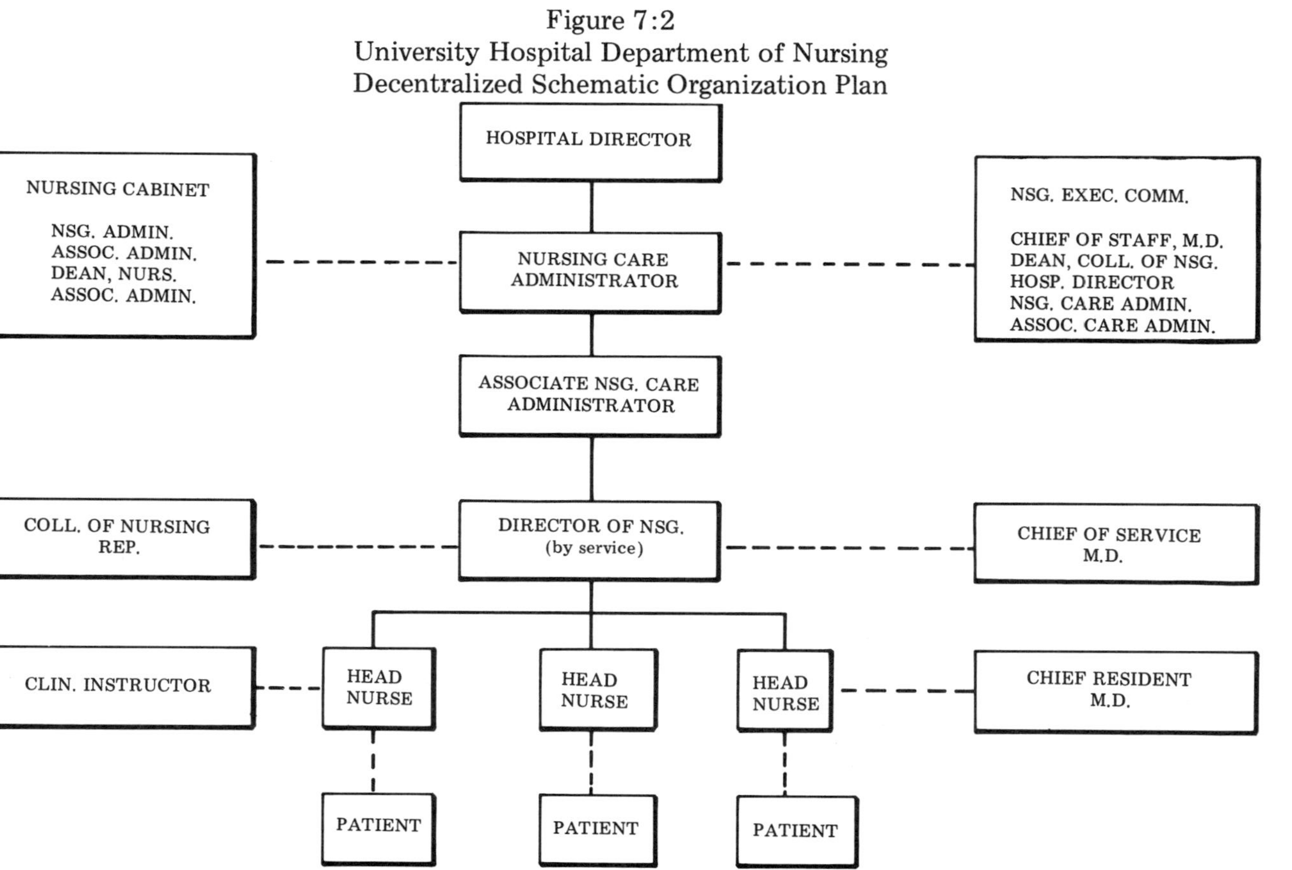

decentralized, care must be exercised to make the transition from one to the other as painless as possible.

In spite of careful planning a change of any magnitude produces some degree of trauma. People don't resist change as much as they resist being changed by others. The nurse manager will do well to help staff members respond to the requirements and risks of change through mutual efforts to treat such requirements and risks as new opportunities for personnel growth and progress. Hirschowitz points to the failure of organizations to appreciate the complexity of human beings and their multiplicity of needs as a contributing factor in lack of adaptation to change.[10] He cites three predictable sequential phases experienced by people going through the transition of change: (1) impact, (2) recoil-turmoil, and (3) adjustment and reconstruction. From experience with systems in transition he suggests what does and does not help ease the difficulty of adjusting to change. Briefly these are:

What helps	What does not help
Involvement in planning and problem solving.	Denial (by those who must face-up to change).
Support and reassurance.	Simplifying complexities.
Guidance.	Overspecializing, by trying to
Presence and proximity of superiors.	overdevelop functions and domains.
Talking about feelings.	Holding on to cherished
Clarification of roles.	habits, routines and rituals.
Respect for values and dignity.	
Hope, through communicative leadership.	

A review of departmental structure can become an occasion for an exciting self-evaluation by each unit and put to work the first item that Hirschowitz identified as helping the change process. One hospital has devised its own self-assessment program that includes having each patient care unit develop its own unit profile. This approach grew out of the collaboration of an associate director of nursing service and a nonnurse with responsibilities in the area of staffing and personnel utilization. They prepared an outline for the content of the profile, with guidelines for its development through the participation of all personnel on the units. Each profile includes the following topics:

1. Description of unit (history, types of patient).
2. Financial status (Budget comparisons, staff understanding and attitude).
3. Quality of care (feedback, audit, opinion polls, incidents, errors).
4. Personnel (age, education, needs, objectives, strengths).
5. Clinical, operational and human resources management (approach, relationships).
6. Inservice education (activity, needs, hospital-wide involvement).
7. Interdepartmental relations (supportive services).
8. Medical staff (attitudes, expectations, rationale).

With the involvement and participation of every person who works on a unit, it is easy to see how this approach applies nurse manager concepts and principles. More than this, the project becomes a self-development and growth process for every member of the unit patient care team. It opens the door to requests for input and help from other departmental and institutional resources, ranging from inservice education to the business office and from the personnel department to other supportive services.

Figure 7:3 provides an example of a program performance plan in which we are involved as part of assisting one university hospital's department of nursing to meet its own particular needs for the future. This plan is included as a pertinent example of how a director of nursing administration can effectively use a nurse management consultant in restructuring a nursing department to meet patient care and organizational goals. The three-phase plan is designed to build upon the existing structure and strengths; facilitate the change process through a maximum degree of involvement of nursing staff members, medical staff, the college of nursing and other resources in the university setting; introduce the problem-oriented system; and strengthen the nurse managers' use of the managerial functions, techniques and skills.

MOTIVATION, POWER AND CHANGE

Nurse managers are no strangers to the exercise of power. You, like everyone else, have been subjected to power in a variety of forms all of your life. And nurses as a group have been discovering ways of exercising power to achieve goals important to them. No extended examination of power and its uses is possible here. But a brief review is pertinent.

Rollo May points out that power is the ability to cause or to prevent change.[11] There is potential power and latent power. Influence is a

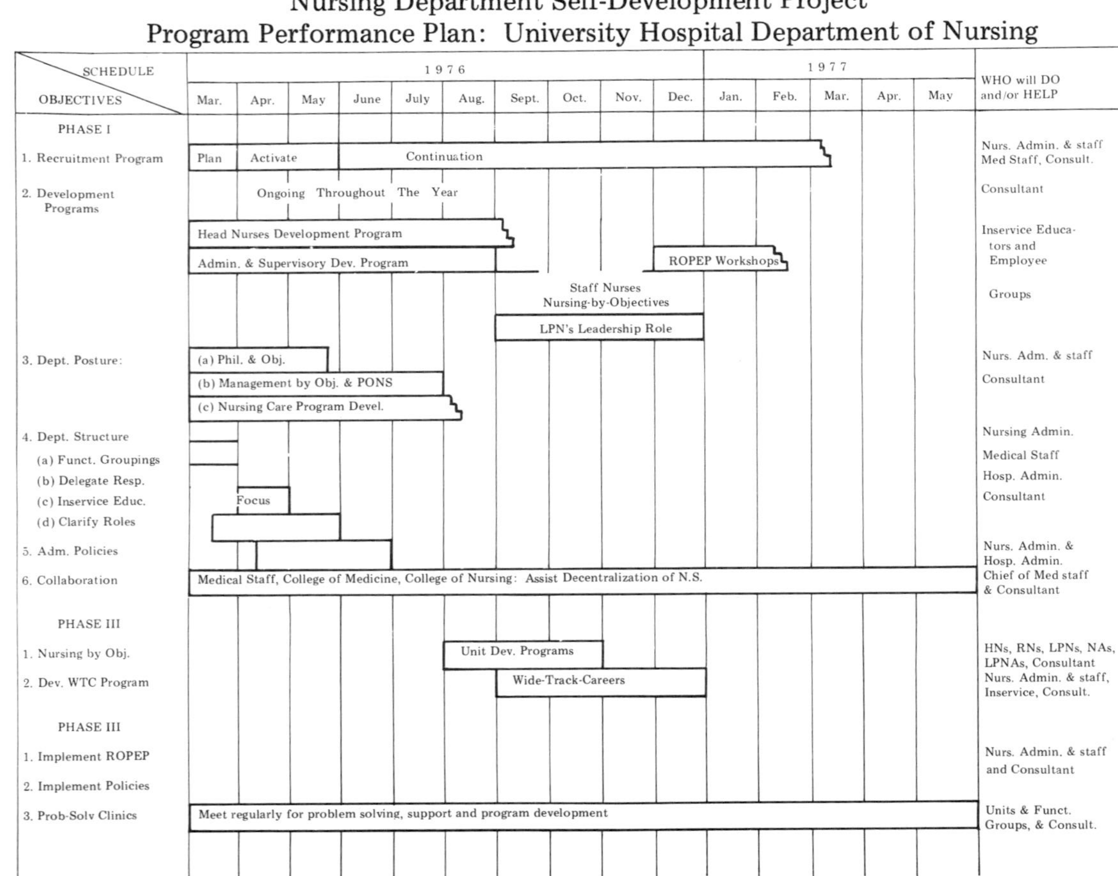

Figure 7:3
Nursing Department Self-Development Project
Program Performance Plan: University Hospital Department of Nursing

form of power. Power may be exploitative, as in using force to destroy choice. Power is competitive and may pit one person against another, productively or unproduct ively. Power is also manipulative. To the extent that this means skillfully to handle or control others, or to influence or manage others shrewdly or deviously, some nurse managers will believe that manipulation is motivation. In a limited sense this is true, because manipulation can cause the self-motivation of others so that they will do what you want them to do. The crux of the matter has to do with the manager's value system as well as the relevancy of the aims in terms of patient care needs and the needs of the person being manipulated or coerced through whatever uses of power.

Adolf Berle, Jr. writes about power from the viewpoint of political science and economics.[12] He points out that power in any form implies at least two relationships: (1) the relationship of the individual or group with the power to the individual or group over which the power is exercised; and (2) the relationship of the particular power organization to the concurrent social-political structure. Little imagination or experience is required to relate these two considerations to the hospital and community environment with the diverse power groupings (political, medical, educational, administrative, managerial, labor union and others) all having an impact upon individuals and groups.

The exercise of power requires organization plus the capability of delegation. The greater the power, the more is the need for delegating. Organization is essentially the mechanism by which decisions and instructions of a central individual or group can be made causative at distant points of application. Building an organization involves gaining and redistributing the power of individuals, a process permitted by the individuals for the benefits they obtain from the group activity.

Berle cites also the internal and external aspects of power. Internal power is that which the central group wields over individuals within the organization and those dependent upon them. The external aspect of power has to do with the capacity to affect others not part of the organization itself. Once again the implications are many for the hospital and nursing organization as related to nurse managers, employees, patients, families and the assorted community groups.

Some understanding of power and its uses is important to nurse managers who are part of, and affected by, organizational power structures. James and Marge Craig offer another view of power as a positive natural force. Their idea of synergic power offers individual nurse managers and other people a way to generate creative cooperation in their personal relations, organizationally, and on a society-wide scale.[13] The book shows how people can move away from mistrust and manipulation and begin to transform strangers or enemies into friends and allies. The Craigs build heavily upon Maslow's concepts to develop a simple and useful motivational model. The authors postulate that when a motivating gap is generated in a person, motivated instrumental behavior will normally follow. This is akin to the earlier section of this chapter in which use of a motivational factors sheet for each of your staff members is suggested. Nurse managers will find the Craigs' book especially helpful. Its thrust is suggested by the authors' use of a quotation from Albert Camus: "Ends do not justify means, but rather means justify means, and means have a way of becoming ends, so it is well to be scrupulous and uncompromising as to means."[14]

MOTIVATION AND ASSERTIVE BEHAVIOR

Robert E. Alberti and Michael L. Emmons provide a definition of assertive behavior in their book *Your Perfect Right: A Guide to Assertive Behavior* as "that behavior which enables a person to act in his own best interests, to stand up for himself without undue anxiety, to express his honest feelings comfortably, or to exercise his own rights without denying the rights of others."[15] The authors clarify nicely the distinction between nonassertive, aggressive and assertive behavior. Nonassertive behavior is characterized by inhibitions, holding in your true feelings, being anxious and hurt, emphasizing your own inadequacies (real or presumed), not striving for your goals, letting others make decisions for you, and general dissatisfaction with the outcomes of your involvement with others. Aggressive behavior is characterized by extreme self-assertion, putting down others, hurting others while making choices for them, disregard for others' worth as persons, and achieving your goals at the expense of others. Assertive behavior is characterized by appropriately expressive, self-enhancing action; choosing for yourself; feeling good about yourself; and usually achieving your self-determined goals.

Table 7:1 summarizes the characteristics, feelings and consequences that are typical for persons whose behavior is nonassertive, aggressive or assertive. The chart also shows how such behavior is likely to affect others. Note that with nonassertive and aggressive behaviors, only one of the two persons involved is likely to achieve his or her desired goal. But using assertive behavior, both persons are likely to achieve their own goals.

Here are examples of three conversations, each exhibiting a different kind of behavior for handling the same situation. As you consider these interchanges, relate what you perceive to Table 7:1.

Table 7:1
Comparative Chart of Behavior Characteristics*

Nonassertive Behavior	Agressive Behavior	Assertive Behavior
Characteristics and Affect on Self[1]		
Self-denying	Self-enhancing at expense of another	Self-enhancing
Inhibited	Expressive	Expressive
Hurt, anxious	Depreciates others	Feels good about self
Allows others to choose for him	Chooses for others	Chooses for self
Does not achieve desired goal	Achieves desired goal by hurting others	May achieve desired goal

Nonassertive Behavior	Aggressive Behavior	Assertive Behavior
Characteristics and Affect on Others[2]		
Guilty or angry	Self-denying	Self-enhancing
Depreciates other person (1)	Hurt, defensive, humiliated	Expressive
Achieves desired goal at other's (1) expense	Does not achieve desired goal	May achieve desired goal

(1) Self, the initiator of the action.

(2) Other(s), the responder to the action.

*This table is adapted with permission from Robert E. Alberti and Michael L. Emmons, *Your Perfect Right: A Guide to Assertive Behavior,* 2nd ed. (San Luis Obispo: Impact Publishers, Inc. 1974), p. 11.

Situation: Insufficient linen has been delivered from the laundry for today's needs on the unit. More linen must be obtained to permit completion of AM care for patients. You call the laundry.

(First interchange, nonassertively.)

UNIT SEC'Y: "Joe? Hey, we're short of linen up here on Three West today. I've got to get some more somehow. Here's what I need...."

JOE: "Now wait a minute! Why are you calling me now? You know it's after 9 o'clock. When did you find out you are short?"

UNIT SEC'Y: "Just a little while ago. The staff is upset and blaming me. Can you help me?"

JOE: "Well, it's probably your own fault. I can't help you now; too busy. Try some of the other floors."

(Second interchange, aggressively.)

HEAD NURSE: "Joe? You've let me down again. We're short today, and we couldn't check it out earlier because you delivered too late. We'll make out OK, though, if you'll have six bed sets available for me in fifteen minutes. I'll send Jack down for them."

JOE: "Darn it all, how can I do that? Two other units want more today too. I'm up to my ears...."

HEAD NURSE: "Look, I don't know about them, but you know we don't hoard the stuff up here. And we've just about had it with your slow delivery. Jack will be down soon."

JOE: "Don't blame me for the delivery schedule. We've got problems with the help I get. If my budget was what I asked for you'd get your linen."

HEAD NURSE: "So what else is new? We still have to get what we need for the patients. But all right, I'll go easy on you. I'll get by with five sets — no less! Don't let me down."

JOE: (sigh). "Don't do me any more favors. Have Jack here in twenty minutes." (Slams down receiver.)

(Third interchange, assertively.)

UNIT COORD: "Good morning, Joe. How's things in your sweatshop?"

JOE: "Lousy. Everybody wants everything two hours ago. So what's your problem?"

UNIT COORD: "Wouldn't you know, we had a few extra admissions and we're caught short. On top of that, I gave two sets yesterday to the second floor. I've got to have six sets, pronto."

JOE: "Have you checked with Four East?"

UNIT COORD: "No. I thought I'd better consult you first."
JOE: "O.K. Have Jack pick up three sets here in ten minutes; then I'll be able to tell him where to get the other three."
UNIT COORD: "Thanks, Joe. You're a gem!"

If you put yourself in Joe's position, you can imagine how he feels in response to each of the three approaches he experienced. You can visualize also the results of each of the three types of behavior exhibited. A short summary of the evidence and the results might be as follows. The letters P, A, and C are included in parentheses to add a consideration of TA in each interchange.

First interchange
Evidence of Behavior:
Unit sec'y (*C*, nonassertive). Here's what I need. Can you help me?"
  Joe (*P*, angry, depreciatingly): "Why are you calling me now! It's probably your own fault."
Results:
  Unit sec'y's goal: Not achieved. No linen from Joe.
  Joe's goal: Achieved. He avoided the extra bother.
Second interchange
Evidence of Behavior:
  Head nurse (*P*, aggressive): "You let me down again. You delivered too late. I'll go easy on you. I'll get by with five."
  Joe (*P*, denying, defensive): "How can I do that? Don't blame me. If my budget was what I asked for...."
Results:
  Head nurse's goal: Achieved (partially).
  Joe's goal: Not achieved.
Third interchange
Evidence of Behavior:
  Unit coord (*A*, assertively): "We're caught short. I've got to have six sets."
  Joe (*A*, self-enhancing): "Have you checked 4 East? Have Jack pick up three. I'll tell him where to get three more."
Results:
  Head nurse's goal: Achieved.
  Joe's goal: Achieved.

"TO BE, RATHER THAN TO SEEM"

The Latin phrase *Esse Quam Videri*, "To be, rather than to seem," appears on the Great Seal of North Carolina and expresses an ideal or goal that must have been in the mind of its original author and in the minds of those visionary men who adopted it for the state. "To be"—to exist in actuality, have reality or life—rather than "to seem"—to give the impression of being, appear—we admit a liking for the value concepts implicit in the motto. The values we associate with the motto have to do with being a genuine person rather than a phony, open and honest rather than closed and devious, trusting rather than suspicious, creative and child-like at times rather than rigid and nonresponsive to the people and wonders around us.

The motto captures in its simplicity much of Maslow's philosophy and humanistic psychology that was his life. Yet Maslow recognized the fact that progress is seldom, if ever, all sweetness and light. In *Eupsychian Management* he described how good eupsychian conditions may produce in some people a regressive, masochistic or self-defeating tendency.[16] When their organization or department is in transition from an authoritarian structure and style to a more participative one, some people do not know how to handle the new freedom situation. The lifting of the rigid restrictions of authority may cause some chaos and release of hostility. It takes some time to convert and retrain authoritarian nurse managers. While this is taking place, some people may view changed behavior by their nurse manager as a form of weakness and attempt to take advantage of the situation. If managers and staff are not prepared for the transitional recoil-turmoil period that involves some disappointment, the temptation will be great to give up and change back to the authoritarian style before the accommodation and acceptance phase of change has been reached. Maslow, sought out by great numbers of people for counsel, had unvarying words of advice about values and goals, "Be stubborn!" This advice has served us well, as it has so many persons whose lives he touched during his lifetime and whom he continues to influence through his voluminous writings in which he shares himself so freely. We can do no better than to pass along to you that same advice.

Consider another recommendation in connection with motivational management. Just as you give attention to developing individualized patient care plans, so should you devote as much attention to individualized employee care plans. After all, patient care plans must be effected by employees whose own morale and motivation have a major influence upon the quality of patient care being delivered. Your role in identifying employee needs and in providing the opportunities for employees to meet their needs, and secure satisfaction-through-the-work-itself, is your surest route to meeting patient care goals.

NOTES

1. M. Scott Myers, *Every Employee A Manager* (New York: McGraw-Hill, 1970), p. 2.
2. Frederick Herzberg, B. Mausner and B. Snyderman, *The Motivation to Work* (New York: John Wiley & Sons, Inc., 1959).
3. Colin Wilson, *New Pathways in Psychology: Maslow & the Post-Freudian Revolution* (New York: Taplinger Publishing . Co., 1972), p. 140.
4. Peter F. Drucker, *Management: Tasks, Responsibilities, Practices* (New York: Harper & Row, 1974), Chapter 23.
5. M. Scott Myers, op. cit., p. 1.
6. Abraham H. Maslow, *Eupsychian Management: A Journal* (Homewood, Ill.: Richard D. Irwin and The Dorsey Press, 1965), pp. 17-33.
7. John F. Mee, "Changing Concepts of Management," *S.A.M. Advanced Management Journal,* 37, 4 (October 1974) p. 22-34.
8. Janet Kraegel et al., *Patient Care Systems* (Philadelphia: J.B. Lippincott Co., 1974), p. 7.
9. Marvin Weisbord, "Why Organization Development Hasn't Worked (So Far) in Medical Centers," *Health Care Management Review 1, no. 2 (Spring 1976), p. 26.*
10. *Notes & Quotes,* July 1974 (Hartford: Connecticut General) excerpted from an article by Ralph C. Hirshowitz in *Personnel,* May-June, 1974.
11. Rollo May, *Power and Innocence: A Search for the Sources of Violence* (New York: W.W. Norton, 1972), p. 99.
12. Adolf Berle, Jr., *Power without Property: A New Development in American Political Economy* (New York: Harcourt, Brace & World, Harvest Books, 1959), p. 79.
13. James H. and Marge Craig, *Synergic Power, Beyond Domination and Permissiveness* (Berkeley: ProActive Press, 1974).
14. Attributed to Albert Camus in the epigraph of James H. and Marge Craig, op. cit.
15. Robert E. Alberti and Michael L. Emmons, *Your Perfect Right: A Guide to Assertive Behavior,* 2nd ed. (San Luis Obispo, Calif.: Impact, 1974), p. 2.
16. Abraham H. Maslow, *Eupsychian Management: A Journal* (Homewood, Ill.: Richard D. Irwin, Inc. and The Dorsey Press, 1965), p. 43.

SUGGESTED READINGS

Books

Alberti, R.E. and Emmons, M.L. *Your Perfect Right: A Guide to Assertive Behavior*, 2nd ed. (San Luis Obispo, Calif.: Impact, 1975).

American Hospital Association. *Employee-Labor Relations in Health Care Institutions*. (Chicago: American Hospital Association, 1975).

National Commission for Study of Nursing and Nursing Education. *An Abstract for Action* (New York: McGraw-Hill, 1970).

Bry, Adelaide. *The TA Primer: Transactional Analysis in Everyday Life* (New York: Harper & Row, Perennial Library,1973).

Craig, J.H., and Craig, M. *Synergic Power: Beyond Domination and Permissiveness* (Berkeley: ProActive Press, 1974).

Drucker, Peter F. *The Age of Discontinuity* (New York: Harper & Row, 1968, 1969).

Goble, Frank. *The Third Force: The Psychology of Abraham Maslow* (New York: Grossman Publishers, 1970).

Hersey, Paul and Blanchard, Kenneth H. *Management of Organizational Behavior: Utilizing Human Resources*, 2nd ed. (Englewood Cliffs, N.J.: Prentice-Hall, 1972).

Jongeward, D. and James, Muriel. *Winning with People: Group Exercises in Transactional Analysis* (Reading, Mass.: Addison-Wesley, 1973).

Jourard, Sidney. *The Transparent Self* (Princeton: Van Nostrand, Insight Books, 1964).

Kraegel, Janet et al. *Patient Care Systems* (Philadelphia: J. B. Lippincott, 1974).

Maher, John, ed. *New Perspectives in Job Enrichment* (New York: Van Nostrand Reinhold, 1971).

Maslow, Abraham. *Toward a Psychology of Being* (Princeton: Van Nostrand, Insight Books, 1968).

Journal of Nursing Administration. *Motivating Personnel and Managing Conflict: A Journal of Nursing Administration Reader* (Wakefield, Mass.: Contemporary Publishing, 1974).

O'Neil, Nena and George. *Shifting Gears* (New York: Avon Books, 1975).

Perls, F.S. and Heffertine, R.F. *Gestalt Theory: Excitement and Growth in the Human Personality* (New York: Julian Press, 1951).

Renders, Thomasino. *Motivation: Key to Good Management* (New York: AMACOM, 1974).

Samples, B. and Wohlford, B. *Opening: A Primer for Self-Actualiza-*

tion (Menlo Park, Calif.: Addison-Wesley, 1975).

Selye, Hans. *The Stress of Life* (New York: McGraw-Hill, 1956).

Terkel, Studs. *Working* (New York: Pantheon Books, 1974).

Toffler, Alvin. *The Eco-Spasm Report* (New York: Bantam Books, 1973).

Wilson, Colin. *New Pathways in Psychology: Maslow & the Post-Freudian Revolution* (New York: Taplinger Publishing Co., 1972).

Articles

Anders, Robert L., "Matrix Organization: An Alternative for Clinical Specialists," *Journal of Nursing Administration,* 5 (June 1975), pp. 11-14.

Charns, Martin, "Breaking the Tradition Barrier: Managing Integration in Healthcare Facilities," *Health Care Management Review* (Winter 1976), pp. 55-67.

Ciske, Karen, "Primary Nursing: An Organization that Promotes Professional Practice," *Journal of Nursing Administration,* 4 (January-February 1974), pp. 28-31.

Fagin, Claire M., "Nurses' Rights," *American Journal of Nursing,* 75 (January 1975), pp. 82-85.

Ganong, Warren L. and Joan Mary, "Good Advice: Motivation and Innovation—Concerns for Nursing Administration," *Journal of Nursing Administration,* 3 (Sept.-Oct., 1973), pp. 7-9.

Ganong, Warren L. and Joan Mary, "Good Advice: Organizational Barriers—Real or Imagined?" *Journal of Nursing Administration,* 4 (January-February 1974), pp. 7-8.

Ganong, Warren I. and Joan Mary, "Good Advice: Patient Care Coordinators," *Journal of Nursing Administration,* 2 (September-October 1972), p. 9.

Hohman, Jo, "Accountability: What It's All About," *Hospitals,* 49 (March 16, 1975), pp. 145-150.

Johnson, G. Vaughn and Tingey, Sherman, "Matrix Organization: Blueprint of Nursing Care Organization for the 80s," *Hospital and Health Services Administration* (Winter 1976), pp. 27-39.

Kalisch, Beatrice and Philip, "A Discourse on the Politics of Nursing," *Journal of Nursing Administration,* 6 (March-April 1976), pp. 29-34.

Maas, Meridean; Specht, Janet; and Jacox, Ada, "Nurse Autonomy: Reality not Rhetoric," *American Journal of Nursing,* 75 (December 1975), pp. 2201-2208.

Monthey, M. "Primary Nursing Is Alive and Well in the Hospital," *American Journal of Nursing,* 73 (January 1973), pp. 83-87.

Chapter 8
Labor Relations and Nursing Management

This chapter and the one that follows will help you develop your own answers regarding your leadership responsibilities in respect to labor relations and personnel motivation. These subjects are vital to your third major area of responsibility as a nurse manager—namely, the managing of your most important resource, your people. We provide some workable, tested guidelines for effective labor relations based upon an understanding of people and their motivation. Labor relations is, after all, people relations—person-to-person relations. This is just as true in employee care as it is in patient care.

"Labor relations" in popular management usage denotes the responsibilities and activities related to maintaining a work force of hourly-paid employees within one corporation, healthcare agency or industry group. Usually the connotation is that of a union-management relationship formalized by a contractual agreement reached through collective bargaining, with all of its attendant implications, requirements and mystique. For better or for worse, nearly all segments of the healthcare industry have been caught up in learning about, fighting off, coping with or adjusting to the labor relations of the 1970s.

How did this happen? It came about largely through the kind of employee relations and managerial leadership practiced in healthcare agencies during the 1960s, 1950s and earlier decades. Individual agencies have remained union-free or have become unionized as a result of their response to the impact of the variety of factors—economic, cultural, political, community, environmental—that influence every institution. This will continue to be true in the years ahead.

What is the current posture of your agency or organization? If you are union-free, does administration welcome the prospect of dealing with one or more labor organizations? Does administration vigorously resist organizational efforts? Or does administration passively accept the seeming inevitability of future unionization? If you already have one or more labor organizations representing employee groups, how does this fact influence administrative leadership? How is your administration's philosophy reflected in policies and procedures? How do these affect your own attitude and actions, and the managing of your department? This chapter will help healthcare agency department heads, supervisors, nurse managers, administrative staff and members of boards of governance consider such questions and their implications for patient care and agency goals. Such searching inquiry, combined with skillful use of the human and technical modes of managing described herein, will contribute to giving positive direction to your own — and your agency's — future.

"Labor relations" (or "industrial relations"), as already described, usually refers to all of the responsibilities and activities of management in maintaining an hourly-paid work force represented by a labor union (the bargaining agent). "Labor relations" may be used less precisely to refer to the broad field of personnel management as it applies to the labor force even when the employees are not members of a labor union.

In this chapter the term "employee relations" refers to the nurse manager's responsibilities and activities in maintaining either a unionized or nonunion work force in a specific healthcare agency. Our reasons are:

- "Employee" is an accurate term for every person on the agency payroll.
- It carries no negative connotations of rank or separateness — of being a group apart from management.
- It is a singular term referring to one person at a time, not to the amorphous group of personnel.
- Employee policies and practices apply to all persons on the agency payroll, with or without a labor union.
- Employees are motivated one at a time, individually, to act as they do.

These reasons are important to us and we hope important to you, for they relate directly to the content and message of this book. Our focus is on management as it applies to the coordination of human effort, of people working together as individuals to achieve common goals for mutual benefit. This kind of management, as previously emphasized, is the process of getting the right things done at the right time through and with the right people.

Our emphasis on the employee as an individual does not preclude a recognition of the fact that people in groups often respond to stimuli and behave in ways that are different from the ways the same persons might respond singly and apart from the group. Nurse managers need to recognize this fact and prepare themselves to provide leadership for groups as well as for people as unique individuals. For this reason we have included in this chapter the "Manager's Guide to Group Relations." It will help you understand some of the special characteristics of groups and how to cope with them.

THE 5M FORMULA

Every manager wants to do a good job. Our experience indicates that healthcare agencies are especially fortunate in having so many well-motivated department heads and nurse managers. And these leaders seem to want to learn more of the art and science of managing.

The 5M Formula is a simple way of looking at the function of a manager in any kind of an organization or department. This formula shows how the combinations of manpower, materials, machines and management provide varying levels of patient care results. The word "formula" is one we would not ordinarily use in connection with the practice of management, since we believe that managing-by-formula is likely to be more mechanistic than humanistic. The best managers use an effective combination of the human mode and the technical mode. Thus "formula" is used herein with its meaning of a symbolic representation, a model, an equation showing some logical relationships. With this in mind, let's examine the 5Ms.

Three of the Ms are arranged to show them in the form of simple addition, each being added to the other to get a result (R):

$$M + M + M = R$$

This shows a combination of manpower, materials, and machines (equipment) that added together in suitable combination produce a result that may be measured and evaluated. R may be reported as number of patient days of care, number of laboratory tests or X rays per day, pounds of laundry per week, meals per month or whatever units are appropriate. And it may be logical to assume that changing the input by some measurable amount will have a corresponding influence upon the amount of output. Thus if manpower (number of hours of work/day by nurses on a unit, for example) is increased by 20%, we might expect to provide care for more patients, or provide more complete services for the same number of patients. The revised formula might look like this:

$$M^{(+20\%)} + M + M = R^+$$

If disposable dishware and utensils are introduced in food service, then less dishwashing might reduce workload and personnel in the kitchen (but with other effects in other departments):

$$M^{-2} + M^- + M^- = r$$

Similarly, other changes in one or more elements of staffing, supplies, equipment, procedures, facilities and so on can be expected to influence results in some predictable way. But every experienced manager knows it's not that simple. It's not that simple because at least two influential elements have not been included in the formula up to this point. One of these is management. This is the department head, the head nurse and all of the supporting supervisory and administrative staff who plan, coordinate and implement whatever happens. So the big M is the manager — you:

$$\underline{M}(M + M + M) = \underline{R}$$

Note that $\underline{M}$-for-manager is shown not just as another addition to the formula but as a multiplying factor. The manager's influence on results is pervasive; it permeates everything else, magnifying the outcomes — usually for the better, sometimes not. The comparison might be shown as follows, using units of 2 for each element in the formula. Example A shows the result if the affect of the manager were nothing more than to add the same amount of input units (2) as the other three M elements. Example B shows the greater result (12 instead of 8 units of output — quantity/quality measures) when the effect of a competent manager becomes a multiplying factor.

Ex. A:	Mgr.	+	Mpr.	+	Mat.	+	Mach.	=	R
	2	+	2	+	2	+	2	=	8

Ex. B:	Mgr.	(Mpr.	+	Mat.	+	Mach.)	=	R
	2	(2	+	2	+	2)		
	= 2	x		6			=	12

But with a less capable manager (a factor of 1 instead of 2) results show as follows.

Ex. A: 1 + 2 + 2 +   2   =   7

Ex. B: 1 (2 + 2 +   2)

        =1 x   6   =   6

The influence of the manager — symbolically as shown above, and realistically in day-to-day on-the-job practice — is profound.

There is yet another M — Money. It is an implicit and essential part of all elements in the formula. We include the financial component as follows:

$$\overset{\$\ \$\quad\ \$\quad\ \$}{M(M\ +\ M\ +\ M)}\ =\ \overset{\$}{R}$$

Money, therefore, ultimately must be included as the least common denominator, the bottom line on the agency's financial statement for the month and year that tells the end result of operating the institution in measurable input/output terms — especially when reported as cost/patient-day. Other output reports are essential too. These are the outcomes in human terms — the quantity/quality/personal data that identify how well the agency is fulfilling its human-service goals. Are these more important than the financial measures? The answer to this is not yes or no, because the question is misleading. Both are essential — the money and the service to people. One does not exist without the other. Adequate financing and a controlled budget are essential if services are to be provided — at any level of quality and quantity.

Some organizations have been experimenting with the human resources accounting method which translates into dollars the human resources of the organization, described and introduced by Rensis Likert.[1]

Admittedly, some managers are better than others in getting the maximum units of service (quality and quantity) out of each dollar of operating expense. One of the reasons for this is their skill in group relations. Group relations has to do with the human factors as they exhibit themselves in group behavior. The following pages examine the characteristics of people in groups and develop the ways to maintain productive group relations.

People in groups are made up of individuals — each with his own skills, values, knowledge and motivation. Each individual person is all-important. Remember, however, that each agency employs several, perhaps hundreds or even thousands, of employees. Each healthcare agency is actually a community. People live there nearly one-quarter of their lives. They must talk with others. They work with a partner or as part of a team. They may eat in the agency too. And they joke and play there too. Our modern agency employees are a far cry from the solo practitioners plying their trades alone. They are part of a healthcare community.

What does each individual look like as part of the agency community, the agency society of which each employee is a part? Each person is one of a group. In its simplest meaning, a group is merely two or more persons who for some reason or other happen to be together. Nurse managers want people to be associated together in such a way that the resulting group meets a purpose and insofar as possible, does so effectively. A group in the healthcare industry, therefore, whether it be the state hospital association, the agency itself, the patient care committee, the planning department, housekeeping, personnel, or the noon-hour luncheon group, is more than merely a number of isolated individuals. Every member of a group has something in common with other members of the group. This common interest is usually the achieving of the group's purpose.

DEFINITION OF A GROUP

A group is a combination of individuals of similar interests who seek personal satisfaction through organized activity. This definition is sufficiently broad that we can use it to apply to any group. The personal satisfaction that comes from being a part of a healthcare agency (or a labor union) is in part measured by the economic and service justification of the agency (or the union). The organized activity is, of course, the method by which the agency (or union) is organized for the effective operation of the agency, society or community (or union).

You live in a world of group activity. You have only to see the damaging effects of a strike of doctors, nurses, or other groups or of a fire in the plant of one primary producer of supplies or the withdrawal of malpractice insurance by a national insurer to see how interdependent is one industry group on the other. Within one agency, the same holds true. If purchasing does not get needed materials on time, if staffing can't supply the needed employees, if the laboratory does not have reports available before they are needed in the OR, or if any other of the many major groups does not do its part, all of the others will suffer.

Each of you fits into one or more of such groups. You cannot escape; you are all members of several groups. There was once a college professor who decided to disassociate himself from all groups. He resigned from his job, his clubs, fraternities, and even the church. After going to great length to become an individual, he found that he still belonged to the human race (he had a life membership in that) and he was a member of a small family group. He had no desire to resign from either. It is evident that most of your life is spent working or playing, inside the agency and out, with groups of members of groups. Actually, you spend most of your hours awake working or associating with others who share with you some similar interests.

Nurse managers can see that it is only through the groups with which persons work that they can satisfy the basic needs and desires which they have as individuals. It is through each person's group activity — through his association with others — that the satisfaction of needs and desires will result. Each person must satisfy many needs and desires through someone else.

But a group is not just a number of isolated individuals. In healthcare, a group is an association of people who by their combined efforts develop a greater effectiveness than the sum of the efforts of each individual separately. By group action, the combined result can be made greater than the sum of the individual parts.

When you examine the individual persons in the group, you see the same things as when you examined them individually — skill, knowledge, values and motivation. There is no reason to feel that individuals will change these when they join a group. However, when you look at the group, or at several groups, the first thing of note is that there are many different kinds of groups — the kinds which make up teams, associations, clubs, committees, unions, families, religious sects, audiences, federations, races, nations, conferences and so forth.

Within the healthcare agency there are many types of groups — administration, middle management, the medical staff, nursing, maintenance, dietary, housekeeping and so on. A second feature we see is that persons, while a part of several groups and loyal to them and their objectives, are still individuals. As both individuals and group members, their own interests and desires may not always coincide with those of the groups to which they belong. In each group we see individual persons. They, as individuals, are separately interrelated with the rest of the group. This can be identified as the Individual-Group Relation.

Listen to one such person, a nurses' aide. Note the relation of this worker's individual interests to those of various groups to which he or she belongs, and note the large number of different groups identified.

Nurses' Aide (proudly): "I've been working in this department for twelve years, and there's no finer bunch of people. I wish we had a team like this running the union. They wouldn't cross us up the way those people do now. (Cautiously) Uh, oh—there's another new aide today. That's the third one they've replaced this month. I'd better watch my own step and not grab too much overtime. Those folks in personnel don't want us to get any time-and-a-half pay. (Pause) (Friendly) Hiya, Jane! How'd you like the way that son of mine played ball at the high school Saturday? Sure put the family name in the news."

Note this worker's pride in the work group, fear for own security, antagonism to personnel department and pride in family group.

Similarly, there must be relations among the several groups. Recognizing the dependence in today's society upon intergroup activity, consider some of these intergroup relations as exhibited in the following comments:

Department head (complaining): "You people up there in the systems office always want us to change our procedures. We're out here on the firing line where the care is actually given. What do you people know about our operations?"
Licensed Practical Nurse (off hand): "We don't want any clinical specialists on our unit. They don't think the way we do!"
Mother (to husband): "I don't think we should let Junior play with those families down by the railroad tracks. Why don't you introduce him to those nice folks you ride to work with?"
Nurse on nights (with envy and feeling of injustice) "Those people on days always have more help. On this shift Louie, Alice, and I have to manage on our own."

In examining any group, you see still further that there are certain individuals who stand out from the rest. These are the leaders, the Group Representatives such as union stewards, department heads and others. Listen to what some group representatives sound like:

The Community Fund Campaign Chairman (helping the group):
"We've got to meet our quotas, folks, and you're the ones who have to do it. I'll give you all the help I can, but the real job is up to you."
Senior Nurses' Aide on evenings (challenging a newcomer):
"What do you want to do, bust up a good thing? I've been on this job three years, and the others and me aren't going to have any young squirt come in and try to show us up with all your eager-beaver stuff."

Union Treasurer (persuading member): "Sure, you have to pay your dues on time; I can't finance you, and the local can't back you with national headquarters. Better let me have the twenty bucks now."

There is still another feature about every group. Each group has certain characteristics. They give it a sort of personality. These characteristics are common to all groups, though they vary in degree with each specific group. The Rotary Club begins a luncheon program with joint singing; a church service ends with the benediction; employee groups are identified with distinctive uniforms. You can name unique characteristics of your own groups. These will be examined shortly.

You have now looked at agency employees as individuals and as members of groups. How is it possible to improve people's relations to the various groups with which they come into contact? This can certainly be done with the individual agency group by setting a pattern of cooperative group action, by understanding the different groups of our agency, by noting the relations of the individual-group conflicts, by spotting the intergroup relationships, by properly working with group representatives and through an appreciation of the general characteristics of groups.

By these means, group action can be improved and employees can be assisted to meet their basic needs and desires. If you inform employees, train them and match them to suitable jobs, you will be increasing their value and stature in the organization. Through this individual and group action you can help employees become more of what they want to be. And if you provide and develop people of greater stature (of greater value) for the 5M Formula, you will (in order to keep your equation balanced) obtain a greater R, the more fully adequate patient care services you would like to provide. By increasing the value of your people (input), you have increased your output.

GROUP RELATIONS GUIDE

The Group Relations Guide Sheet (see Exhibit 8:1) provides a summary of some of the key points in the foregoing pages, expands the information about group relationships with additional facts about groups, identifies important general characteristics of groups and then gives useful guides to managerial action in relation to groups. It deserves your careful reading, understanding, and application.

As you examine the guide sheet, consider its validity in the light of your own experience with or understanding of union-management

Exhibit 8:1
Group Relations Guide Sheet

PART I

Good group relations is more than the absence of conflict; it is a positive condition of mutual reliance which the manager must build.

THE MANAGER'S FORMULA FOR GROUP RELATIONS

A. UNDERSTANDING *m.b.* TOLERANCE ———→ AGREEMENT

B. RESPONSIBILITY *m.b.* COORDINATION + INCENTIVE ———→

COOPERATIVE ACTION

---

m.b. = modified by   ———→ = leads to

BASIC NEEDS AND DESIRES OF INDIVIDUALS

1. Survival
2. Security
3. Social (Love and Belonging)
4. Status (Self-esteem, pride)
5. Self-actualizing

SCIENTIFIC APPROACH TO MANAGEMENT PROBLEMS

1. State or isolate problem
2. Get facts
3. Restate problem
4. Analyze
5. Take action
6. Follow up

These are satisfied through group activity. Earning the respect and confidence of all groups is the life blood of group relations.

THE COMMON AIMS OF EVERY GROUP

1. An economic order favorable to the attainment of its objectives.

2. Cooperation, natural or imposed, of other groups in the attainment of its objectives.

3. The right to utilize its skills to the greatest advantage.

4. The maximum amount of freedom in the exercise of its skills.

5. A maximum return for the skills of its members.

The violation of accepted common law principles of justice in handling group relations is a manager's most fatal error.

PART II

GROUP FACTS	MANAGER'S ACTION

A. DIFFERENT GROUPS

1. People belong to several different groups.	1. Identify his different groups and those of the people with whom he deals.
2. There are organized and unorganized groups.	2. Change unorganized groups into organized working teams.
3. There are friendly and hostile groups.	3. Create friendly working groups.

B. MAN-GROUP RELATIONS

4. Group members have individual desires.	4. Harmonize members' individual desires with those of the group and vice versa.
5. Members move from one group to another according to satisfaction received.	5. Make his group an "in group" for its members.
6. Group membership results in conflicting loyalties.	6. Reduce (as far as possible eliminate) conflicting loyalties in members.
7. Groups are not always satisfied with their members.	7. Fit himself into his groups. Select members that fit and help them fit.

C. INTERGROUP RELATIONS

8. Conflict and antagonism among groups defeat groups' purposes.	8. Strive for cooperative action by all groups.
9. In intergroup conflicts, people align themselves with the group of which they feel most strongly a part.	9. Align himself (get others also to align themselves) with group whose objectives offer greatest long-term benefits.

D. GROUP REPRESENTATIVES

10. Effective group activity requires group leadership.	10. Lead his group and help representatives of his subgroups to be leaders.
11. Group follows its representative only when feeling he works in group interest.	11. Stress interest in group to which he and his members belong. "Be on their side."
12. Most management groups comprise representatives of other groups.	12. Apply same principles and formula as to any other group.

GENERAL CHARACTERISTICS OF GROUPS

1. Group members will fight and sacrifice for their group and its objectives so long as the group serves its members.
2. Groups respond to emotional appeals.
3. Selfishness is dominant in group objectives.
4. Groups use distinctive methods and techniques.
5. Group thinking is simple Land direct and may be more accurate than that of individuals.
6. Group effectiveness varies with the degree of intragroup balance.
7. Group effectiveness varies with the degree of active participation by group members.

relations. Labor unions exist because they fulfill needs — people's needs. Healthcare agencies exist also to fulfill needs — people's needs. When the methods of meeting people's needs cause conflict, at least part of the reason may be identified in the group relations guide sheet. Appropriate action by nurse managers can help prevent or mitigate the results of such conflict.

Nurse managers and other leaders have a responsibility, as noted in Chapter 1, to learn and use management terminology that is precise and appropriate. There is a distinction, for example, between a *complaint* and a *grievance*. A *complaint* is anything which is brought to your attention, or which you observe or sense, which is a possible cause for dissatisfaction, or unfair treatment (real or imagined) or an employee. A *grievance* is a formal complaint presented in accordance with the provisions of the labor agreement (the union contract with the employer); or, in nonunion situations, based upon a violation of established personnel policies, and presented in accordance with a published grievance procedure.

You can usually decide whether a complaint is a genuine grievance by asking yourself two questions:

1. Did the employer violate the contract? If the answer is yes, you've got a grievance.
2. Has the worker been treated unfairly by the employer? If the answer is yes to this question, you've probably got a grievance, even though you're not sure that the contract has been violated. Sometimes this kind of grievance is hard to win, though, because of a loophole in the contract.

Usually a grievance is a violation of the contract. You may not think so at first, but if you read your contract carefully you can usually find some section of it that deals with the kind of problem your grievance involves.

"Complaint" is the broader term which can be used for all causes of dissatisfaction. Thus in the remainder of this chapter "complaint" is used as the all-inclusive term for complaints and grievances in both union and nonunion agencies. " Grievance" is used herein only in the meaning of a violation of the labor contract between the employer and the union.

It should be kept in mind, however, that "There is in plain fact, nothing wholly predictable — nothing cut and dried — about what takes place in situations of actual or impending conflict. Both responses and outcomes are various."[2]

THE NURSE MANAGER'S ROLE IN COMPLAINTS

A complaint is not a threat. It need not be a problem. The most experienced nurse managers look upon a complaint as an opportunity. A complaint provides an opportunity for the nurse manager to:

1. Understand the reasons for the complaint. What's the real human basis for this complaint?
2. Evaluate the substance and value of a complaint. Has the employee been treated unfairly? Has there been a violation of agency or departmental policies?
3. Develop a consistent positive approach to the handling of complaints. Am I avoiding the danger of locking-in too soon?
4. Consider, in every complaint situation:
   a) The objective in handling it.
   b) The attitudes involved and their influence on the participants.
   c) The facts and assumptions involved.
   d) The relative costs resulting from the alternative courses of action which are possible. What should I really want to achieve, and what are the alternative ways I can do it?

Your success in helping successfully to resolve complaints is directly related to your ability to: (1) view a complaint as an opportunity for improving communication with your people; (2) avoid getting mad or disconcerted when you are presented with a complaint; (3) see how each complaint can lead to greater understanding, rather than be a chance to engage in a boxing match; and (4) avoid the danger of locking-in too soon; and make commitments only after checking feelings, facts, policies and past practices.

Much may depend upon your own leadership style. A review of the brief discussion of leadership styles in Chapter 1 is relevant now in connection with the foregoing aspects of handling complaints. For example, think about a recent complaint with which you were involved. Was it yours to handle? Do you feel you had the responsibility and authority to deal with it? What needs were in evidence—the employee's and yours? What assumptions did you make? What was your objective? Recall the facts, attitudes and feelings as you identified them. What was the cost of that complaint? Was it a problem or opportunity? What were your feelings? Did they help or hinder a successful outcome?

Cost of complaints that turn into grievances can be great. Some of the costs are direct and measurable and may be hundreds or thousands of dollars if arbitration is involved. Other costs are indirect, but expensive nonetheless in terms of group relations, motivation and impact upon patient care services. Arbitration is a method of settling a dispute through recourse to an impartial third party whose decision is final and binding. Arbitration is voluntary when both parties of their own volition agree to submit a dispute to arbitration. It is compulsory when the two parties involved are required by law to submit the dispute to arbitration. Arbitration, costly yet sometimes justified, may be the end result of negligence by the nurse manager when a complaint first comes to light. The best time to resolve any complaint is when it is first made by an employee to the nurse manager. Thus our emphasis is upon ways to minimize the causes for complaints (through progressive policies, procedures and management); to treat each complaint seriously and expeditiously when one occurs (resolving it fairly between employee and the nurse manager whenever possible); and if further steps are necessary, to resolve the complaint justly without arbitration.

Exhibit 8:2 presents a summary of a complaint that became a grievance which went to arbitration. It provides a typical example of the frustrating, lengthy, time-comsuming, costly involvement of many people trying to resolve a case that, on the face of it, seemed to deserve a decision to support the Hospital's position. The arbitrator's award may have been wise and just; it's difficult to evaluate as just or not by the time the final decision is made. Sometimes the nature of the complaint itself seems to have changed because of all that happens in the often lengthy interval between initial complaint and the ultimate arbitrator's decision. The message is clear. To minimize the frequency and cost of complaints you can provide progressive leadership, minimize the causes for job dissatisfaction, maximize the conditions that lead to job satisfaction, build effective work teams using your understanding of group relations, focus on human needs and patient care goals and resolve complaints promptly.

When your job requires your involvement in handling grievances, an excellence reference book is *Grievance Handling: 101 Guides for Supervisors* by Walter E. Baer. It presents the grievance machinery as "the formal process, preliminary to any arbitration, that enables the parties to attempt to resolve their differences in a peaceful, orderly, and expeditious manner."[3] It includes among the 101 guides some

Exhibit 8:2
THE FALSIFIED RECORDS ARBITRATION
The Confidential Case File on Millie Arnold
Case Number 292

The Grievance:

Grievance No. 127 was filed October 26, 1974 by Millie Arnold, and read in part as follows:

Nature of Complaint—"I was unfairly terminated on Rules of Conduct No. 26 which states, 'Deliberately falsifying employment records or other records such as time tickets or patient charts.' I am asking to be reinstated with pay for lost time as I am not guilty."

The Issue:

Was the discharge of Millie Arnold for just cause?

The Hospital Position:

The Hospital contends that the discharge was for just cause because the grievant deliberately falsified the record of her tardiness on Friday, October 20, 1974 and was properly discharged for violation of Rule #26 following a fair and objective investigation establishing the misconduct.

The Union Position:

The Union contends that the grievant was the victim of harassment and discrimination; that the discharge was not for just cause, and requests her reinstatement with full seniority.

The Award:

The grievance of Millie Arnold is sustained to the extent that the penalty of discharge is reduced to disciplinary suspension with loss of seniority beginning October 25, 1974 and ending as of the first payroll period following April 25, 1975, at which time she shall be reinstated in a position equivalent to the one she held on October 25, 1974. She shall retain all seniority earned prior to October 25, 1974.

The Reasoning:

The full opinion and award of the Arbitrator in this case, and the other related papers which describe the development of the grievance, total twenty-seven pages. They reflect the employee's record of former disciplinary actions for the same and similar infractions in the past two years. She appears to be a satisfactory worker when on the job. This arbitrator decided the award as stated, in spite of a decision to terminate another employee in an almost identical arbitration case a year previously.

helpful management suggestions for supervisors, a 50-item leadership checklist, what followers look for in a leader, and related tips on discipline and training.

PROCEDURE FOR HANDLING COMPLAINTS

An effective five-step procedure for handling complaints as opportunities is:

1. Let the employee talk
   - Listen to the employee in private. Put the employee at ease. Allow the employee plenty of time to tell the story. Don't interrupt. Keep your temper.
   - Get all the details. Identify opinions and feelings.
   - Make certain the real complaint is the expressed one.
   - Repeat the complaint in your own words. State the opinions and feelings. Arrive at a common understanding.
   - Tell the employee when you will give an answer.

2. Check the facts (including opinions and feelings)
   - Investigate the employee's story. Gather all the details you can about the complaint.
   - Refer to agency and department policies and past practices (precedents).
   - Know the employee and his needs.
   - Consult with others whose experience, knowledge or observation may aid you in arriving at a decision.

3. Arrive at decision (considering alternative courses of action)
   - Based on facts (including opinions, emotions, feelings); and agency and department policy, procedures, and past practices.

4. Tell the employee the decision
   - Plan when, what, where and how you are going to tell the employee.
   - If complaint is justified, admit it graciously.
   - If complaint is unfounded, explain why.
   - Don't be bulldozed.
   - If the decision is adverse to the employee, prepare the case for possible appeal.

5. Follow through
  • Take prompt action to correct the cause of complaint.
  • Check with the employee to see that the complaint has been eliminated.

This procedure is one which has been developed from the experiences of successful supervisors and managers, and also, as you can see, from a much older procedure, the scientific method in problem solving:

1. State the Problem (Put it in writing).
2. Collect Facts, Opinions, Feelings (Recognize your assumptions).
3. Analyze the Facts (Redefine the problem).
4. Develop Solutions (Consider the alternatives).
5. Take Action (Be clear and direct).
6. Follow Through (To assure expected results).

The use of the 5 steps in handling complaints helps prevent the temptation to give snap decisions, to take action precipitously, to let a complaint drag along or to do those other human things that allow a complaint to fester, become a grievance, and turn an opportunity into a real problem for you.

FACTS, INFERENCES AND DECISIONS IN PROBLEM SOLVING

Good judgement requires careful distinction between two kinds of ideas we have about the world around us. Such ideas stem from our observations and inferences. Observations are products of personal experience. To observe something we must see, hear, feel, smell or taste it. Inferences are decisions about the meanings of our observations. Both kind of ideas are indispensable to our proper functioning; but when we mistake inferences for observations, we have trouble.

You may wish to test your own human tendency to make unwarranted inferences and assumptions. Two exercises, the Bad Judgement Tests in Appendix D, provide such an opportunity. You may be surprised at your own level of assumptions. If you are like most people you won't agree with all of the answers as given for the two exercises. Even after discussion with others you may still be in disagreement, unable to comprehend the reasons for the "?" answers — or even some of the "T" and "F" answers. In fact, you may become upset, mad and hostile. If so, then you have a complaint, but no grievance. The answers as provided are strictly in accord with the contract (the instructions, the "ground rules") provided for each exercise. Perhaps a cooling-off period is needed to permit you to take a fresh look at the exercises and your complaint. Perhaps part of the problem (opportunity?) has to do with an unclear understanding of the instructions and what T, F, and ? mean. If so, then your complaint is a true communications opportunity. These two exercises, like so many simple-seeming complaints, turn out to be quite complex when several persons get involved — with their various levels of understanding, values, motivations, feelings and opinions. The message is clear — use the 5-step procedure with skill and care.

Always be careful with "the facts." The definition of a fact is (1) something having existence supported by evidence, an actuality; (2) truth, reality; (3) an act considered with regard to its legality as in "after the fact." Transactional Analysis (TA) provides a helpful model for keeping facts in their proper place in relation to prejudgements (values, prejudices) and feelings (emotional reactions).

Edwin Bixenstein has written a scholarly and helpful description of "The Value-Fact Antithesis in Behavioral Science." In his introductory statement, Dr. Bixenstein poses a consideration of values and facts in a context that will be helpful to professional nurse managers:

> While values emerge ever more prominently for considera-
> tion in the reflective, scientific literature of our time, a stub-
> born cleavage remains in our construing of values and facts.
> This separation is encouraged by a 19th century construction
> of science which places limitations on humans as scientists, in
> an effort to preserve an unlimited and superhuman concep-
> tion of science. The thesis of this article is that all knowledge
> resides in the human response to events, that this response is
> irreducibly subjective and evaluative, and that facts are a
> special class of (communicated) values distinguishable by in-
> traobserver redundancy and interobserver consensuality.[4]

The article with its generous listing of additional references will be rewarding for those nurses who want to pursue an understanding of the relationship between values and facts in a philosophical, scientific, and humanistic manner. As the author says in his summary comments, "Realism invites us to relax, to be both human and scientist."[5] Exactly! That is our theme in this book. The many nurse managers we know are — or want to be — both human and scientific in their contributions to patient care management.

USING TRANSACTIONAL ANALYSIS (TA) IN HANDLING PROBLEMS AND COMPLAINTS

A transaction occurs whenever you are involved with someone else. TA is a way of analyzing, understanding and improving your interactions with others. TA provides a simple way of talking about the complexities of human interaction based upon the study of ego states exhibited by human beings. This is explained in a very few words and many pictures by Adelaide Bry in *The TA Primer*.[6] The author says everyone has three buttons inside them all the time waiting to be pushed. These are the PAC buttons:

(P) stands for the parent in you.

(A) stands for the adult in you.

(C) stands for the child in you.

You need all three of the PAC buttons. When you learn to push them selectively, on purpose, rather than randomly and irrationally, your results usually will be better. You will be able to give different strokes to different folks. And you find yourself in the happy situation of "I'm OK, You're OK." A variety of good books on TA are available in paperback editions. We suggest *The TA Primer* because it is so brief and easy to understand.

The usual approach in solving problems is to get facts about the problem situation, review the facts logically to identify the causes of a problem, then decide what action should be taken. This rational adult (A) approach is shown simply as follows[7]:

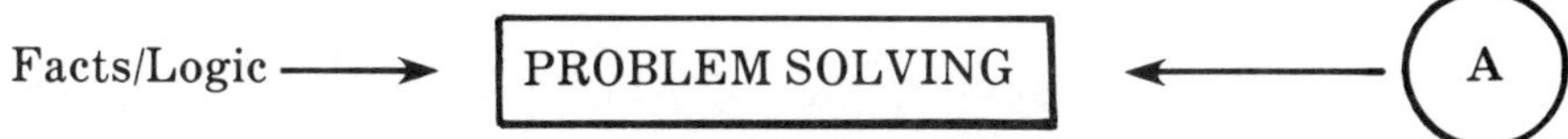

The experienced problem-solver recognizes a difficulty. People involved with a problem often are very emotional about it. They may ignore the facts. They let their feelings get in the way. They act more like a child (C) than as an adult:

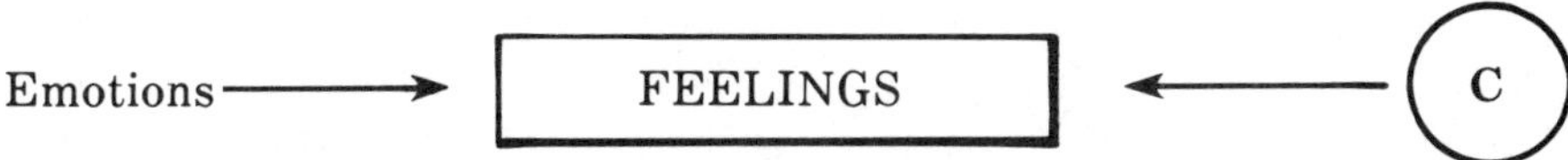

In addition, people often allow their prejudgments to affect their thinking. ("What can you expect from a person of that race, religion or sex?" Or, "That's wrong." Or, "You should never do that." Or, "Listen to me; I know best.") Prejudging a situation or person comes out of one's apperceptive mass. For better or worse, it reflects a lifetime of shaping one's values, beliefs, morals, and prejudices. It is the parent (P) in action.

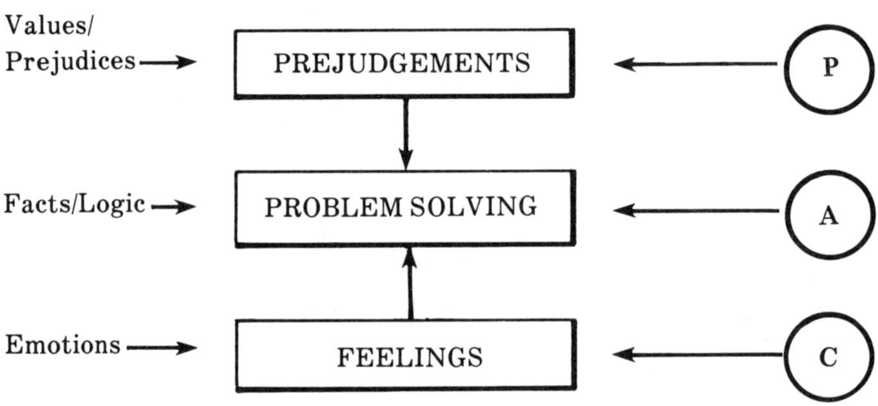

Every person has some of the parent, adult and child in his personality. Some persons maintain a reasonable balance of P, A and C. Others allow one to predominate, and seem to react consistently as P, A or C. Recognizing this fact is helpful in your involvement with others, in solving problems, handling complaints and in getting good results.

As you read more about TA you will learn how you can handle certain kinds of transactions that cause problems.

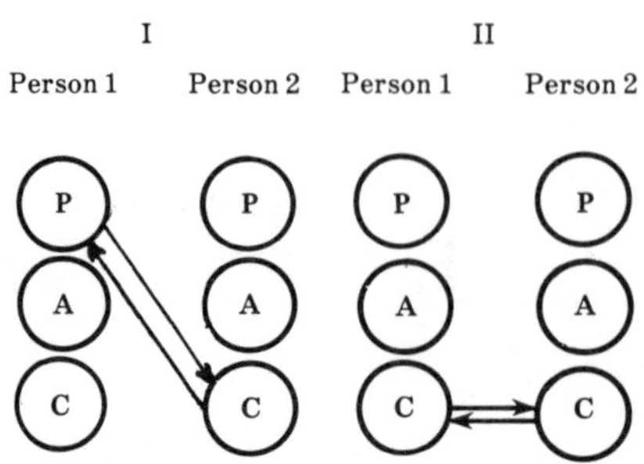

Examples I and II show complementary types of transactions. They may sometimes reflect a kind of game-playing, but are not so likely to cause the difficulties of Example III.

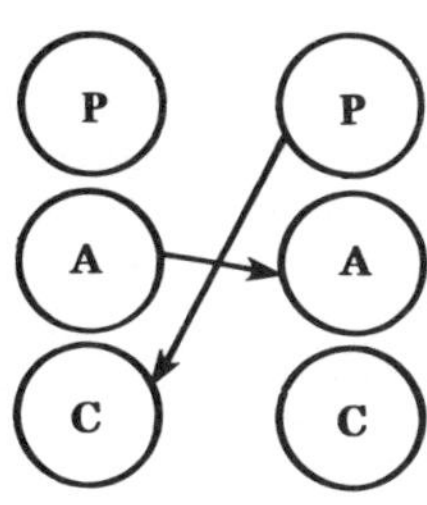

Crossed transactions cause problems. For example, in example III you may be Person 1 calling the food service department to ask, as one adult to another, "Will Mrs. Foster be able to have her special diet tray at 11:30 A.M.?" Person 2, in the kitchen, replies (from her parent), "Listen, Kiddo, we'll deliver what's ordered. We don't need any checking from you." This kind of crossed transaction is ready-made for fireworks. It should put up a warning sign to you: Danger Ahead—Proceed With Caution.

We know a fine operating room head nurse who learned TA and began to try it with the surgeons. She had always been accustomed to playing her parent (or tearful child) to the surgeon's emotional child and found her role demeaning and frustrating. At first, when she tried to change the relationship to that of adult to adult, she used the language of TA and didn't succeed. But when she learned to stay in her adult role and not talk about it, just use adult behavior, it worked. She is justly proud of having been able to bring about an adult-to-adult relationship with the surgeons. In fact, she is now the OR supervisor.

As a nurse manager you observe and get involved in many kinds of transactions each day. You can enhance your value as a facilitative helper as you recognize P or C buttons (yours and others) being pushed at the wrong time and find ways to help untangle the crossed transactions. Such perception and skill will greatly enhance your ability to resolve complaints and grievances.

SKILLS AND TECHNIQUES IN EMPLOYEE RELATIONS

There are a variety of managerial skills and techniques, involving both the human and technical modes, that are necessary in carrying out your employee relations responsibilities as part of your management functions of planning, doing and controlling. A technique, of course, provides a model which can be used repeatedly to aid in achieving your objectives. A skill is something you do with your head, hands or body to carry out a technique. Here is a listing of some managerial techniques and skills you may use in carrying out your employee relations responsibility.

Techniques

- Handling Complaints
- Group Negotiation
- Management by Objectives
- Results-Oriented Performance Evaluation
- Transactional Analysis
- Wide-Track Career Planning
- Critical Incident Technique
- Crisis Intervention
- Third-Party Intervention
- Managing Change
- Securing Involvement

Skills

Communicating (behavior, body language, eye contact, facial expression, listening, reading, silence, speaking, touching, writing)
Conceptualizing
Decision making
Problem solving
Instructing
Day-to-day coaching

Techniques are likely to be only as good as the skills of the people who use them. The personal values and motivation of the manager have great influence upon the use of the skills and techniques. Your workworld as a healthcare manager is ultimately no more nor less than you choose to make it—for yourself, your employees and your patients.

In our view, you are the key person in your employee relations situation. This is because you are the Big M in the 5M Formula. You have no need for gimmicks, crash campaigns, devious strategy or behavior modification techniques for influencing employees. Progressive, business-like, humanistically oriented management is needed to permit and facilitate the need satisfaction of employees so that their self-motivation is meshed with agency goals.

THE ROLE OF THE NURSE MANAGER IN NEGOTIATIONS

When a bargaining unit is first established, there is a tendency for much time and effort to be expended by all concerned in we/they, win/lose interchanges. We have observed that this carry-over from the initial negotiating effort evidences itself in hospital settings in ways that are counterproductive in terms of patient care. The newly awarded contract often weighs heavily as a stinging defeat to management and as a sweet victory to the bargaining unit members. The intricate ploys in the serious game of the unionizing effort give way to the newly imposed rules and regulations established by the contract. The hours once devoted to the strategy of winning or losing the election are replaced by hours involved with the shop steward in union member problems, grievance procedures, living up to the letter of the agreement, educating all concerned in understanding and living within the contract, dealing with violations of the contract, and to preparing for the next contract negotiations.

It is an exercise in futility for managers to maintain an attitude of hostile, controlled acceptance of the bargaining unit and for unit members to demonstrate smugness. The critical issues have been decided. The healthiest attitude is to accept that fact and move toward developing positive relationships, healing old wounds, and working together. Accomplishing such a feat is easier said than done. The impact phase of this change from nonunion to union status within a department of nursing will begin to give way to a recoil/turmoil phase and eventually lead to acceptance, accommodation or continued rejection by the individuals involved.

Once a bargaining unit is a reality, the role of the nursing administrator has several facets. The first of these is that of maintaining a facilitative leadership role in blending the contract provisions into the goals and objectives of the department of nursing. It is vital that the nursing administrator accept and not abdicate responsibility for sound management decisions. The nursing administrator and nurse managers at all levels within the department must deal openly with employee complaints and grievances as they arise. This is simply what nurse managers have been or should have been doing in the absence of a union.

Two major changes occur with the advent of the union contract. First, the nurse managers have an additional set of rules and guidelines which must be followed in handling grievances. These new rules are contained in the legal document which is the union contract. Secondly, the employee group is emboldened and empowered to pursue what they see as new expectations and rights which formerly may have received less-than-satisfactory attention in their view.

This combination of the contract provisions and the new feeling of group solidarity and power among the work force may cause the nursing administrator and nurse managers to feel that they have lost status, authority and control. Such will be the case only if they permit it to happen. In some instances, whatever feeling they had previously of status, power and influence may have been misplaced or misused. In these cases the union serves to bring about a more equitable relationship, the kind of participation and involvement achieved by the goal-oriented manager even without third party intervention. In other situations where capable nurse managers or administrators experience a diminution of their management responsibilities and rights, adequate support and advice by the hospital administrator (or his counsellors) can aid in renewing and maintaining the feeling of position, responsibility, and authority that is justly deserved.

It is pertinent to review once again the workworld of the nurse manager. You remain the center of your workworld. What you know and how you feel has much to do with how you act and react. If you overreact to a significant change in your work environment—namely, the new presence of the union—then it may be because of a distorted perception of the influence of the union on your actions. You remain the manager with the same scope of legitimate functions. Necessarily, however, you must adapt to the new element in your workworld, the union. In many ways this is little different from your adapting to nursing audit, medicare documentation requirements, patients' rights, and similar regulations affecting healthcare management in your agency.

Another responsibility of the nursing administrator is careful preparation for contract negotiations. It is wise to go to the bargaining table well prepared to bargain in good faith about issues of major concern to management and employees. This means having facts and figures to support opinions and proposals. An informed forecast of the probable demands that will be brought to the bargaining table by the union representatives will permit preparation for a strong bargaining position. Management should not place itself in the position of simply receiving the union demands and responding thereto. Rather, management should prepare its own bargaining proposals for presentation to the union. The nursing administrator can be an important contributor to such proposals. One example of such action was a group bargaining situation in a mid-western city which resulted in establishing a three-month residency for recently graduated nurses with a new starting rate lower than the prior minimum rate for graduate nurses. This could not have happened without the initiative of the nursing administrators who worked together and bargained in good faith to secure it.

The goal-oriented nursing administrator wants what is best for the healthcare agency, the patients who are the recipients of care and services, and the nursing personnel who provide that care and service. Such an administrator goes to the bargaining table prepared to secure the best contract for all concerned.

NOTES

1. Rensis Likert, *The Human Organization* (New York: McGraw-Hill, 1967).
2. Harry and Bonaro Overstreet, *The Strange Tactics of Extremism* (New York: Norton, 1964).
3. Walter E. Baer, *Grievance Handling: 101 Guides for Supervisors* (New York: American Management Association, Inc., 1970), p. 3.
4. Edwin Bixenstine, "The Value-Fact Antithesis in Behavioral Science," *Journal of Humanistic Psychology,* 16 (Spring 1976), p. 35.
5. Bixenstine, ibid., p. 55.
6. Adelaide Bry, *The TA Primer: Transactional Analysis in Everyday Life* (New York: Harper & Row, Perennial Library, 1973).
7. For this adaptation of TA to problem-solving we are indebted to Dr. Fred Biamonte, of the Graduate School of Pace University in New York.

SUGGESTED READINGS

Books

American Hospital Association. *Employee-Labor Relations in Health Care Institutions* (Chicago: AHA, 1975).

Baer, Walter. *Grievance Handling: 101 Guides for Supervisors* (New York: American Management Association, 1970).

Bry, Adelaide. *The TA Primer: Transactional Analysis in Everyday Life* (New York: Harper & Row, Perennial Library, 1973).

Dougherty, James. *Union-Free Management and How to Keep It Free* (Chicago: Dartnell Corp., 1968).

Ganong, Joan and Warren. *HELP with Labor Relations through Motivational Management* (Chapel Hill, N.C.: W.L. Ganong Co., 1976).

Gellerman, Saul W. *Management by Motivation* (New York: American Management Association, 1968).

Goble, Frank. *Excellence in Leadership* (New York: American Management Association, 1972).

Harris, T.A. *I'm OK—You're OK* (New York: Harper & Row, 1967).

Health Law Center. *Nursing and the Law* (Germantown, Md.: Aspen, 1975).

Herzberg, Frederick. *Work and the Nature of Man* (Cleveland: World Publishing Co., 1966).

Jongeward, D. and James, Muriel. *Winning with People: Group Exercises in Transactional Analysis* (Reading, Mass.: Addison-Wesley, 1973).

Likert, Rensis. *The Human Organization* (New York: McGraw-Hill, 1967).

Maslow, Abraham. *Eupsychian Management: A Journal* (Homewood, Ill.: Richard Irwin, Inc. and The Dorsey Press, 1965).

Nierenberg, Gerard. *The Art of Negotiating* (New York: Cornerstone Library, 1968).

Myers, M. Scott. *Every Employee a Manager: More Meaningful Work Through Job Enrichment* (New York: McGraw-Hill, 1970).

Stagner, R. and Rosen, H. *Psychology of Union-Management Relations.* Behavioral Science in Industry Series, edited by Victor H. Vroom. (Belmont, Calif.: Brooks/Cole Publishg Co., 1965).

Render, Thomasino. *Motivation: Key to Good Management* (New York: AMACOM, 1974).

Rutter, William A. *Labor Law,* 2nd ed. (Gardena, Calif.: Gilbert Law Summaries, 1974).

U.S. Dept. of Labor. *Important Events in American Labor History 1778-1968* (Washington, D.C.: GPO, 1969).

Chapter 9

Education: The Nurse Manager's Role

Learning and teaching are natural human activities. They are a part of everyday living and they are important components of a problem-oriented nursing system. Everyone caught up in the struggle for health—patients, families, significant others, healthcare professionals and the myriad of related healthcare workers—all are involved in the educational process revolving around the maintenance or regaining of health, the disease process, and even birth and death. There is so much to learn and so much to teach that it comes as no surprise to find education as an essential element in the foundation component of PONS— and as a component in and of itself.

Both teaching and learning are involved in all of the five components that make up the problem-oriented system. The assessment part of the nursing process includes the nurse's learning about the patient and those people important to the patient as well as his problems, needs, and goals. In turn, the patient learns about himself, about illness, wellness, and about the healthcare system. Teaching is an integral part of the implementation phase of the nursing process. Patient and family teaching is built into the planning phase. It follows that the evaluation of results as part of the nursing process is also a time for learning what has resulted for the patient from the planning and doing.

The nursing record and the auditing components of PONS also provide teaching and learning opportunities—by both patient and nurse. During the nursing process, the patient sometimes is the teacher and the nurse is the learner; in other situations during the process, the roles are reversed and the nurse becomes teacher and the patient is the learner.

In a different context this teaching/learning process works in similar fashion for the nurse manager and the rest of the nursing staff. At times the manager is thrust into the role of learner by members of the staff. At other times the roles are reversed and the manager becomes teacher to the staff. This is true at all levels of management from the nurse administrator to the head nurse (or that person's equivalent.)

The process of educating yourself and others is ongoing. It takes place in both formal and informal ways and settings. It happens in offices, classrooms, hallways, elevators, patient rooms, control centers, nursing stations, cafeterias, automobiles, streets. It takes place over the telephone; via tape recorder, radio, television; through the reading of books, periodicals, newsletters, patient records, memos, workbooks; by completing patient data bases and reviewing patient referral forms; through face-to-face conversation, discussion, argument, lecture; in committees, meetings, reports, presentations. Indeed, the nurse manager is bombarded by the educative process at every turn. It is as natural as breathing and just as essential. Since you cannot escape it, the best thing to do is to welcome it as a healthy part of the management process and put it to good use for yourself, your staff, your patients and your colleagues.

Education has both cognitive and affective elements. In the writings of George Brown it becomes abundantly clear that knowledge and feelings are not separate entities moving along parallel paths that never meet or mingle. Brown defines "confluent education" as the flowing together of the cognitive and affective elements in individual and group learning.[1] People have feelings about what they know. Learning is a process that necessarily engages both your emotions and your intellect. Heart and mind, feelings and logic — all are continuously involved in the learning and teaching in which people engage.

Many persons find it easier to identify their thoughts than their feelings. Thoughts seem to relate to facts, to a framework of logic, to a rational relationship of things and ideas we know about. People can cope with matters of logic and usually can fit them comfortably into their own apperceptive mass, the associational area of your brain. But many people find it difficult to identify and cope with feelings. There are a wide range of emotions that people experience. Too often they pass unrecognized. You may feel confused, irritated, angry, amused, anxious, put down, enlightened, wondering, puzzled, excited, apprehensive, expectant, warm, cold, impressed, disaffected, apathetic, inspired, alarmed, thrilled, belittled, provoked, joyful, agitated, happy, sorrowful or whatever. Your emotions, whether among those just listed or others, are all acceptable. They are neither good nor bad. They are simply yours and deserve to be recognized as such. And these emotions influence learning and teaching. This being the case, we hasten to explain a term that may not be a part of everyone's vocabulary.

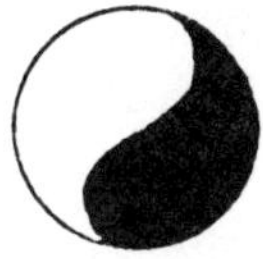

Yin and Yang is the ancient (11 B.C.) polarity theory of two primal forces: the dark and the light, night and day, earth and heaven, female and male, the yielding and the firm. This is symbolized by a circle divided by a thin s-curve in which one side is dark and the other light to show the rotational interplay and flowing together of opposites. Confluent education can be seen as the interplay and flowing together of seeming opposites, the affective and cognitive aspects of the teaching/learning process. Unrecognized or unresolved emotions can affect the learning outcomes in unexpected ways. They can effectively sabotage, even if unwittingly, the best efforts of both teacher and learner—regardless of who may be experiencing the emotions. Or they can be utilized in a positive way, building upon the natural yin and yang relationship of learner and teacher, to achieve the educational objectives of both. There needs to be a careful, appropriate balancing of the cognitive and affective elements of education.

An exceptionally skilled California pediatrician has been discovering for herself something significant about the doctor-patient relationship and its influence upon the healing process. This physician had always assumed that a young patient admitted to the hospital realized it was for the purpose of curing the ailment, whether sore throat or broken leg. But when she began to ask the children themselves why they were in the hospital, she found that they had reasons quite at variance with her beliefs as to why they were there. Some answered, "Because I was naughty." Another said "I stole some money; that's why I'm here." In terms of the newer findings in psychosomatic medicine, those may very well be significant reasons for the illness or accident and subsequent hospitalization, formerly overlooked or not understood by the physician, and hence having an effect upon the healing process or the lack thereof.

It is possible that the teacher/learner relationship in a healthcare setting can benefit from the kind of questioning approach and dialogue experienced by the doctor and her patients. The pediatrician found that when she and her patient became colleagues in healing, the patient recovered faster. There is surely a message here for the nurse in modifying the traditional teacher and learner roles so that the educational process becomes more of a mutual adventure of colleagues in learning.

HUMANISTIC MEDICINE, NURSING, AND TEACHING

One of the more recent trends in healthcare is being identified as humanistic medicine. It applies the precepts and practices of humanistic psychology. One of its hallmarks is an holistic view of the patient. Patients are seen not as the "CVA in Room 428" or the "liver in Room 727," but as the complex human beings they are, with all of their physical, psychological and spiritual components—the yang and yin interplay and flowing together of natural forces, sometimes in seeming opposition to one another. This trend toward humanistic medicine demands the implementation of more humanistic teaching. The holistic approach is not new in nursing. What is new to many nursing educators and managers is the confluent approach to teaching and learning. However, there is an ever increasing trend in nursing programs and healthcare agencies toward a flowing together of the cognitive and affective elements.

ATTITUDES AND VALUES IN PERSPECTIVE

Every nurse is a teacher. The nurse as a good teacher is often characterized by descriptive terms that connote positive attitude, strong sense of values, adherence to principles, vitality, enthusiasm, empathy, understanding of individual differences and thorough knowledge of the subject. Undoubtedly the good learner also can be characterized by the same or similar terms. This matter of attitudes and values deserves further examination. Consider yourself, your contributions, and your opportunities in a broader framework of relationships of self and others in confluent education. You are at the center of these relationships, you and your apperceptive mass, made up of your values, motives, knowledge and skills.

Ornstein attempts to reconcile two basic approaches to knowledge: one, the rational; the other, the intuitive.[2] He explores the bifunctional brain, the differences between the right and left sides, and the psychology of consciousness. Ongoing studies hold considerable promise for greater self-direction and control, with significant implications for confluent education. Dr. Bogen, meeting in December of 1975 with educators from 19 campuses of the California system, emphasized experience as part of the education process. He said, "We have neurologic evidence to favor the view that talking about something and writing about it are very inadequate ways to learn."[3]

TEACHER/LEARNER VS. MANAGER/WORKER

The role of a teacher and the role of a manager (in heathcare, education, business, government and other institutions) have many common characteristics. Both teachers and managers, for example, are responsible for:

- — the persons (students, workers) whom they supervise.
- — setting standards and goals.
- — assigning work to be done.
- — providing suitable supplies, tools, working environment.
- — giving instructions.
- — maintaining discipline.
- — the effective utilization of resources (time, money, facilities, people).
- — carrying out organizational philosophy, objectives, policies.
- — solving problems and conflicts.
- — evaluating the performance of students and workers.
- — recommending advancement as deserved.

The foregoing list provides evidence of the similarity of the roles of teachers and managers. Further examination in depth will demonstrate how the two roles merge in other ways. One of these other aspects of role similarity is the characterization of leadership style. In Figure 3:3 entitled "The Role of the Manager" the left column headed Authority-Oriented lists eight identifiable behavioral patterns for this leadership style. The Plan-Lead -Control diagram shows how this type of manager sees his role in contrast to the employee role of doing the work. In the right-hand column headed "Goal-Oriented" are the same eight aspects of a manager's role, but now stated in behavioral terms that express a subtle but distinct contrast in role concept. The diagram illustrates an expanded job concept for the employee, in which he has greater opportunity to plan and control his work activities in addition to doing the work itself. Now, change the title at the top of the page. Cross out the word "Manager" and change the title to read "Roles of Teacher/Facilitator/Learner." Read again each statement in the left column. Note how closely these same items apply to the traditional authority-oriented teacher. Similarly in the right-hand column, few words require changing (job incumbents to learners) to have the same descriptions apply for the learning facilitator role. The revised diagrams are shown in Figure 9:1.

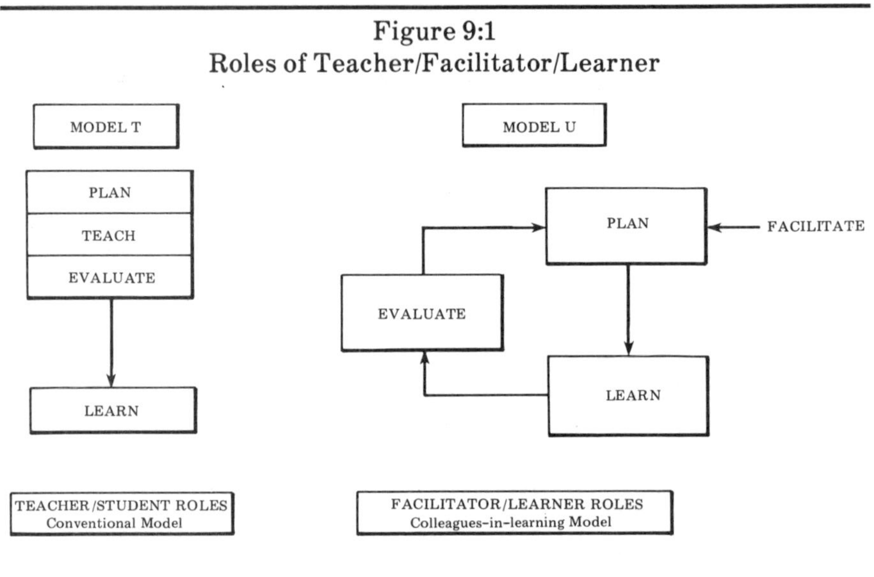

In the Teacher/Student diagram Model T, and the Facilitator/Learner diagram Model U, the letters "T" and "U" are used for several reasons. Visually, the two diagrams can be seen as a T and a U (on its side). And "T" stands for Teacher, the more traditional version. And while the Model T Ford was a great automobile and served its users well in its day, it has long since gone out of style — as have some teaching methods. The "U" represents the full impact of you that goes into the learning-facilitator role in confluent education.

The teacher/manager analogy deserves to be carried one step further. Among the ranks of professional managers, the real professionals are looked upon as those who are skilled developers of people, good teachers. People working with these managers grow and learn. They move up to broader management or clinical responsibilities because their managers have facilitated their growth, have helped them to learn. In a similar vein, the best teachers are likely to be those who are good managers. As such, these teachers make sure that adequate tools, supplies and facilities are available for use by the learners; encourage the learners to set their own goals; give access to information the learners want; aid their self-evaluation; recognize achievement; help the learners build on failures; view themselves as facilitators of the learning process, as colleagues in learning.

Nurses who are in tune with the concepts of goal-oriented management and facilitative teaching can blend the two meaningfully in a patient care setting. Such nurses—in positions of administration, coordination, supervision, head nurse or practitioner—bring to the nurse manager role a truly participative approach to the myriad of problems that must be dealt with daily.

KNEE GROUPS AND EXPERIENTIAL LEARNING

A variety of useful experiential teaching techniques may be used by nurse managers in their learning-facilitator role. One of these is the knee group. A knee group is defined as a discussion group of three to five people seated in a circle of chairs pulled so closely together that the knees of the participants touch. The purpose of such a group is to stimulate the maximum degree of informality and closeness among the participants so that a lively, productive interchange of ideas and feelings can occur in an atmosphere of trust and acceptance.

The knee group as a technique is an outgrowth of the Nurse Manager ACT-U-ARs, which are self-actualizing seminars we designed and conduct to help nurses in management positions sharpen their managerial skills and organizational effectiveness. The technique was utilized first because of the need to divide a workshop group of 30 nurse managers into small discussion groups of four or five in a meeting room with no tables and limited space. The unexpected benefits were so significant that it has since been used repeatedly with similar excellent results, regardless of the size of the room or the number in the total group.

The conference leader first provides a brief explanation of the knee group purpose and procedure. Usually the group members huddle their chairs in small circles so that their knees are in contact. This allows the people to get "in tight, not up tight," to share thoughts, feelings and ideas through intense, personal contact with one another.

The initial response of participants as they begin to form the knee groups is usually one of humorous comments and joviality. The process of arranging the chairs and getting settled provides an opportunity for informal remarks and laughter which appear to relax the participants and ease them into goal-directed discussions.

A typical ACT-U-AR knee group session generally proceeds as follows:

- The group takes a few minutes to get better acquainted.
- A specific exercise, discussion question or topic is agreed upon. The nurses focus their attention on the talking and listening aspects of the communication process. Distractions such as paper, pencils and books are put aside.
- One person in each group volunteers or is selected to serve as recorder and jot down brief notes, when pertinent.
- The seminar leader promotes informality by his own attitude and actions.
- When appropriate, the leader may join a group briefly, getting into knee contact or not, depending upon the situation.
- At the end of the time period, the leader calls a halt to the discussion and takes a few minutes to wean the participants from their intense involvement.
- A spokesman for each knee group then presents the conclusions and salient points developed by each group.
- Additional comments are often volunteered by others in the groups.
- When all groups have reported, the ACT-U-AR leader builds upon the knee group conclusions to reinforce principles and concepts which are basic to effective management in nursing.

Since the inception of the knee group technique several years ago in the ACT-U-ARs, it has been adapted for use in a wide variety of healthcare and educational settings where the focus has been upon newer concepts of management in nursing. Nurse-managers have begun to use the knee group themselves for improving their own communications and problem-solving processes in a variety of settings. Some that have been reported to us include problem-solving by coronary care head nurses with their staff, personnel evaluation discussions by head nurses with staff members, and staff meeting discussions led by nurse administrators. Virginia Gierke, Director of Nursing Service, Memorial Hospital, Menomonie, Wisc., wrote recently:

I have found knee groups very successful in my nursing staff meetings. R.N.'s, L.P.N.'s, Nursing Assistants, CSR. Techs and O.R. Techs are all included. They worked through their feelings about establishing priorities. Some of the feelings many Nursing Assistants and Nursing Staff expressed are:

1. "The patient pays so much per day—he deserves a complete bath everyday."
2. "I just don't see why we can't have more staff—we can never complete all our work."
3. "We just don't have time to work on Nursing Care Plans."
4. "After our work is done there is no time for a patient-centered conference."

In knee groups the following solutions were presented:

1. Start on the patient care plan at the time of admission. Involve the patient and his family in his plan of care.
2. Schedule patient-centered conferences three times a week at least and actively work at establishing priorities in order to find time for this most important part of the patient's plan of care. This will be scheduled early in the day, not after the "work is all done."[4]

Knee groups are a highly effective technique for securing involvement in establishing and achieving mutual goals for the improved management of nursing care and for problem solving. The close contact and intense concentration on matters of mutual concern promote feelings of genuine worth on the part of the nursing staff participants. They feel recognized as concerned persons with ideas and opinions deserving of consideration. Emphasis is upon sharing and experiencing rather than telling. The outcome is better problem definition and improved solutions with enthusiastic follow-through action. Thus knee groups provide a method for the nurse manager to secure wholehearted participation by others in the setting of goals and in implementing programs of managing by objectives.

Success by nurse managers with knee groups requires a basic belief in the worth of each individual and a willingness to perform within a framework of mutual trust and respect. Experience shows that in such a climate the nurse managers can improve team results by having their people get their heads together by getting their knees together.

The use of knee groups is especially valuable in structuring learning experiences that build upon the necessary intertwinement of the cognitive and affective components of the educative process. Following immediately is an example of a set of experiential exercises designed to help participants better comprehend the significance of the five human needs. The experiences are meaningful even when carried out

Exhibit 9:1

Exercises in Experiencing the Human Needs

Time: 20 — 30 minutes.   Group size: Large or small.

Explain that the purpose of this exercise is to permit the participants to feel the needs and their influence on motivation and behavior.

1.   Survival. Ask group to close eyes to minimize distractions. Instruct group, upon your signal, to take a deep breath and hold it for as long as possible. Tell them not to breathe again until you give the signal to do so.

   (Allow 50 — 60 seconds to pass.)

   Ask: —   Why didn't you hold your breath longer?
           —   Why did you breathe again before I told you to do so?
           —   What was your basic need?
           —   What would all of you do if right now this room were sealed and the air extracted from the room?

   Discuss implications. Point out (at this time as well as at end of entire exercise) that the other four human needs can be felt just as strongly, just as biologically, as the imperative need for air.

2.   Security. First select a group member to stand close beside you as you explain this exercise to the group. Lean up against each other slightly, exerting modest pressure. Ask the other person to pull away from you abruptly at some time during your instructions to group.

   Say to group, "Most human beings find security in their relationship to another person. That's just fine as long as the other person is there. But if one loses the support of the other (through leaving home, divorce, death) then one experiences the sense of loss. As is true with other needs, we are not conscious of its importance until it is no longer being satisfied."

   Ask group to stand in pairs, side by side, and experience how it feels when the other removes the support. Allow group discussion of reactions and feelings.

3.   Social: Love and Belonging. Instruct group to sit or stand in tight groups of six or seven persons, arms locked together, with one person on the outside.   The group is to talk together and ignore the outsider completely, while he tries to join the group by whatever means possible.

   (Allow several minutes, calling a halt as soon as appropriate.)

   Allow group discussion of the experience. "How did it feel?" (To group members; to the outsider?) "If you got in (or didn't), how did you do it? What was group reaction?" Comment on the physical and emotional aspects of being an outsider. People must find a way to belong. This unsatisfied need sometimes leads to the formation of other groups, even if made up of the outsiders themselves.

4. Status, Esteem. Instruct group members, in pairs or in knee groups, to tell each other, "What I like about you is . . . ." After a few minutes, when each person has told and been told, allow group discussion. Focus summary on implications for on-the-job employee relations and patient care.

5. Self-Actualization. Describe self-actualization as you understand it—a continuing reaching out for becoming more of what you can be, for peak experiences, for ongoing growth and development of oneself.

    Ask knee groups to share personal examples of their own self-actualizing experiences, if any, as they understand it.

Conclude exercise by relating the experiences to confluent education, patient teaching, and the human and technical modes in patient care.

---

not using knee groups. They carry extra impact, however, and achieve the objectives more successfully when the experiences take place in the small groups and individual reactions are shared and discussed within each group. Your own experimentation with various ways of carrying out these learning experiences will prove exciting and helpful to you in developing your own innovative approaches to carrying out your learning-facilitator role for the maximum benefit of your patients and staff members.

THE UNIQUENESS OF YOUR SETTING

The healthcare facility in which you find yourself is unique. It is the only one of its kind, solitary, sole, single. Its true quality of being the only one of its kind is conferred by the people, like you, who make it come alive. The people make it one of a kind. The same building with different people takes on a whole new character. Even a change of only one key person can influence the organization's personality.

In terms of confluent education, this uniqueness is the sum total of the flowing together of the thinking and feeling of all the people involved in the day-to-day operation of the institution. Your institution and the people involved in it have needs that cry out for innovative teaching techniques which will capitalize on the singular potential within each person—teacher/facilitator, student, worker, patient/consumer.

Innovative teaching in your unique setting calls for varying kinds of knowledge, skill and ability put to use through two basic modes, the technical mode and the human mode. "Mode" refers to (1) A manner, way or method of doing or acting; (2) A particular form, variety, or manner. The technical mode places its emphasis primarily on the techniques, systems and procedures related to nursing, patient care, unit management and teaching. The main emphasis is on things rather than people. The human mode has as its focus the people aspects of caring, planning, problem-solving, organizing, staffing, communicating, teaching and learning. It includes the psychosocial aspects which involve understanding and awareness of self and other, attitudes, values, motivation and personal attributes. The emphasis is on people rather than things.

Since all nurses are expected to be teacher/facilitators, they need to find a way to strike the necessary balance in the use of the technical and human modes in each setting. Both modes are necessary. Neither is independent of the other. They are, and need to be, confluent.

PRINCIPLES OF LEARNING AND TEACHING

There are available some useful roadmaps for the person who sets out upon the pathway to confluent education. These roadmaps are the learning principles, some traditional, others more innovative and in tune with recent advances in an understanding of Homo sapiens. Learning and teaching, you will recall, are two parts of the educational process. For the process to be meaningful, both the learner and the teacher need to share their feelings, skills, experiences and knowledge. Both teacher and learner need to have feedback on their progress.

Consider now some of the more conventional concepts of learning. Margaret L. Pohl's *Teaching Function of the Nurse Practitioner* presents some useful principles as guides to action.

1. *Perception is necessary for learning.*

This principle is pertinent in relation to the discussion of a learner's apperceptive mass in Section 1. People learn by relating new information and teachings to what they already know and have experienced. When experienced teachers say that they must begin from where the learners are, they are saying that they can build upon only what the learners have the ability to perceive; teachers cannot expect students to learn something not perceivable within their individual apperceptive mass. As we will soon see, however, there are ways to increase the ability to perceive, and hence to learn, within the apparent confines of current knowledge and experience levels.

2. *Conditioning is a process of learning.*

Conditioning is the process or result of inducing new or modified behavioral responses. To this extent, conditioning is learning. For example, in learning the Problem-Oriented Nursing System (PONS), it is necessary to become familiar with the five components of the system: The Foundation (Principles of Practice), The Nursing Process, The Problem-Oriented Nursing Record, Nursing Audit, and Education (for Patients and Staff). Students can be helped to learn these steps by:

- Writing them down on paper.
- Pairing off and explaining the steps to each other.
- Going to the board and writing them on the board.
- Repeating the foregoing steps, but including all of the elements for each of the five components of PONS.
- Practicing use of the components.

In such repetitive exercises, supported by suitable rewards and praise, the students remember and learn the PONS components and also the elements of each of the components.

3. *People learn by trial and error.*

Much learning is acquired through trial and error. This method works, often out of necessity. While costly, lessons learned in this way are often valuable. In certain situations where there is the need for immediate learning, such as an emergency, people do the best they can and learn from their doing. Making mistakes and correcting them as they are recognized is also a form of trial-and-error learning. People learn by doing.

4. *People learn by imitation.*

This is certainly one of the most common ways of learning. People tend to emulate and imitate those whom they admire and respect as well as others who have served as role models for them. They play the game of Follow the Leader. This is not just a childhood game, but one played by adults. Your nursing staff, your associates and subordinates, observe you and say to themselves (often subconsciously), "My boss earned his/her job by being the way he/she is, by acting the way he/she does, by thinking the way he/she does. So if I become more like my boss, behaving, thinking, and doing like him/her, then I'll be a success, too." Sobering thought! Yes, people learn by imitation. The power of example is strong.

5. *Developing concepts is part of learning.*

A concept is an idea, especially an abstraction drawn from the specific. Thus a concept is a kind of mental picture a person develops about things in the world around him. This process of conceptualization, of concept formulation, takes place in a person's mind — just as all learning is accomplished by the learner, not the teacher. Thus concepts of a particular technique or nursing procedure may take on different characteristics in the minds of different learners.

For example, terms like "team nursing," "nursing by objectives," "performance evaluation," or "problem-oriented medical record" can mean different things to different persons. Their concepts vary according to how they were taught such techniques and how they have experienced them on the job.

One person's concept of the problem-oriented medical record is an acronym: POMR. Another person may visualize the file folder known as the patient's chart containing the carefully documented components: (a) Defined Data Base, (b) Complete Problem List, (c) Initial Plans, and (d) Progress Notes. A third nurse, however, when conceptualizing POMR, sees a whole system of quality nursing care integrated with medical care by the physician to provide the best possible patient care. A fourth person, a recipient of care, sees POMR as something that means better care for the patient, a shorter convalescence, lower cost and an ongoing, readily accessible medical history of himself. Concepts, like perceptions, will continue to be influenced by the apperceptive mass and motivation of the individual. The cliches, "We see what we want to see," and "We hear what we want to hear," are meaningful. Thus the teacher — as guide, facilitator, and counselor — faces a real challenge in helping learners to conceptualize reasonably consistent ideas about programs, techniques and practices that affect organizational performance and patient care.[5]

SOME NEWER PRINCIPLES OF LEARNING

Carl Rogers in *Freedom to Learn* offers a number of principles (or hypotheses) that he believes can be extracted from current experience and research. These are all related to newer approaches to learning designed to set students free for self-initiated, self-reliant learning. Here are some of his principles:

1. Human beings have a natural potentiality for learning.
2. Significant learning takes place when the subject matter is perceived by the student as having relevance for his own purposes.

3. Learning which involves a change in the perception of oneself is threatening and tends to be resisted.
4. Those learnings which are threatening to the self are more easily perceived and assimilated when external threats are at a minimum.
5. When threat to the self is low, experience can be perceived in differentiated fashion and learning can proceed.[6]

One can grasp quickly where Carl Rogers is coming from. He has over 40 years of experience as a teacher, experimenting and innovating in his approaches to his classroom students. He is renowned as a therapist, with unusual psychological insights and skills. He brings to his book a keen sense of urgency, deriving from his desire to contribute help to teachers and educators in a time of literally fearful crisis and incredible challenges in education. There is much of value for the nurse or teacher in what Rogers has to say. His focus is clearly on learning by doing, experiential learning, confluent education. Such learning is defined as having a quality of personal involvement, being self-initiated and pervasive (affects behavior, attitudes, even the personality of the learner), evaluated by the learner, and having its essence in meaning. This kind of learning requires a different concept of teaching. Rogers offers these precepts:

- Learning is facilitated when the student participates responsibly in the learning process.
- Self-initiated learning which involves the whole person of the learner — feelings as well as intellect — is the most lasting and pervasive.
- Independence, creativity, and self-reliance are all facilitated when self-criticism and self-evaluation are basic and evaluation by others is of secondary importance.
- The most socially useful learning in the modern world is the learning of the process of learning, a continuing openness to experience and incorporation into oneself of the process of change.[7]

THE CLINICAL CONFERENCE AS A LEARNING OPPORTUNITY

The clinical conference offers nursing personnel an opportunity to utilize in the work setting sound principles of teaching and learning. The clinical conference deals with real day-to-day patient-care problems. It has many advantageous features as a learning environment. These features include the immediate nature of the problems and discussion topics, the intense personal involvement, the patient-focused concerns, the caring-sharing-doing tradition and the prospect of personal need satisfaction through participation and successful follow-through action. People want something to happen during, and as a result of, the clinical conference. Such desire, and the realization that each person is expected to contribute to a plan of action and its execution, helps to provide the kind of motivational climate so essential to learning. Conference participation promotes the kind of involvement that helps many persons satisfy some of their felt needs. Because a clinical conference demands participation at both cognitive and affective levels, there is an excellent opportunity for the nursing staff to observe, learn and practice the skills of group leadership and problem-solving.

When patients (clients) are included in the clinical conference, there are benefits to them as well as to the staff personnel. Such benefits include: (1) Pooling of subjective and objective information; (2) Using everyone's creative potential in problem identification and problem solving; (3) Raising of questions that may or may not have immediate answers; (4) New kinds of learning as the patient and staff become colleagues in healing.

Carl Rogers indicates that "we are faced with an entirely new situation in education where the goal is the facilitation of change and learning."[8] If, as Rogers states, the goal of education is the facilitation of change and learning, then the role of the teacher must be modified accordingly. What is now needed is a facilitator of change and learning. Such a facilitator role requires a different attitude and outlook than that of the traditional teacher. Compare the definitions of facilitate and teach. "Teach" means to impart knowledge, to instruct, to cause to learn. "Facilitate" means to make easier; to aid; to assist. The contrast between the two terms is striking. The orientation, the whole way of perceiving the teacher/learner relationship, is altered when the facilitative role is emphasized. This means a modification in how both teacher and learner think of their roles, their relationships, their expectations and their methods of evaluating progress. Some newer techniques and methods are also required, and they are available.

SOME ADDITIONAL PRINCIPLES OF TEACHING AND FACILITATING

There are a number of principles of teaching conceived for the more traditional role concept of the teacher that are still useful and valid. They have served as helpful guides for many excellent teachers. Here are some of these principles:

1. The philosophy of the teacher affects teaching and learning.
2. Teaching requires effective communication and rapport.
3. Teaching requires planning and evaluation.
4. Teaching skills can be acquired through practice and observation.
5. The needs and objectives of the learner, the teacher and the program must be considered.
6. Teaching must be relevant to the learner to be effective.

Every one of these principles is applicable to nurses in their role of teacher for staff and patients. Here are five additional guidelines for learning facilitators:

1. The facilitator has much to do with setting the initial mood or climate of the group or class experience.
2. The facilitator helps to elicit and clarify the purposes of the individuals in the group as well as the more general purposes of the group.
3. The facilitator relies upon the desire of each learner to implement those purposes which have meaning for him as the motivational force for significant learning.
4. The facilitator endeavors to organize and make easily available the widest possible range of resources for learning.
5. The facilitator regards himself as a flexible resource to be utilized by the group.

These guidelines also apply to the nurse as teacher. The difference in emphasis between the two sets of guidelines is apparent. Each reflects a different orientation, a different way of thinking about—and attitude toward—the teacher/learner relationship. Even allowing for differing individual interpretations in what the words and sentences mean, the contrast is impressive.

HELPING THE STAFF TO LEARN

The educational process is an integral part of every nursing department's ongoing functional responsibilities. Over the years the nursing departments of healthcare agencies have created educational departments. These have been given a variety of names—Inservice, Staff Development, and Continuing Education—to name a few. These departments vary in the level of sophistication of their programs, the level of preparation of their directors and staff, their size, facilities, purpose and budget. For some small healthcare agencies there may be one person who has the inservice function as a part of many other responsibilities. Others have centralized the educational function for the entire agency, sometimes under a director of human resources development with a registered nurse as part of the teaching staff. There are all kinds of variations in between those two organizational extremes.

Before exploring ways to organize for the educational function of a nursing department that is supportive of a problem-oriented nursing system, there is a need to clarify some terminology with regard to the functions.

One way to examine the functions is to define them:

"Orientation," as one function, is defined as an organized program to acquaint new nursing personnel with the physical and social environment of the agency, the specific assigned work location and the relationships within this environment of which they are now a part.
"On-the-job Training," as another function refers to that aspect of inservice education designed to help nursing personnel learn, or to improve their performance in doing, a specific task or procedure. It enhances the skill level of the individual.
"Inservice education," as yet another function, is defined as any educational experience that affects the work performance of nursing personnel. The focus is specifically job related.
"Continuing education," as still another function, is defined as organized learning experiences throughout life that contribute to individual growth and development. It is designed to help the nursing staff keep current with new concepts, knowledge and techniques that relate to healthcare and nursing activities.

Each of these functions is appropriate to the role of education in a work setting. In a decentralized nursing department a considerable number of the activities within the first three functions take place at the patient-unit level under the overall direction of the nurse manager (by whatever title). In such a setting every nurse is accountable for the teaching part of his or her job. The nurse manager teaches the nursing staff, the staff teach other staff members as well as patients, families and signigicant others. All learn from one another. Such a setting is ready-made for the use of confluent education principles and guidelines.

Even a decentralized nursing department needs support and assistance from a staff development department (by whatever title). Some aspects of the educational functions are expediently handled by such a department while others rightfully are carried out at the patient-unit level. The following columns provide a typical division of responsibility between the staff development department and the patient care units for the educational functions:

Staff development department	Patient unit

1. For Orientation

- To the agency and nursing department, and the overall organizational structure, philosophy, goals, objectives, policies and rules.

- To the layout of physical facility.

- To the nursing department's patient care program.

- To agency and nursing department systems and techniques.

- To the unit and its specific organizational philosophy, goals, objectives, policies and rules.

- To patients, records, reports.

- To unit personnel, staffing, patient assignments, unit meetings and conferences, performance responsibilities and performance evaluation plan.

- To the unit's physical layout details.

- To the unit's patient care program.

- To the unit's application of systems and techniques.

2. For Inservice

- Plan, organize, coordinate, implement and evaluate.

- Agency and department-wide inservice programs—such as CPR, fire and safety, disaster, new procedures, systems and techniques.

- Clinical conferences of broad interest to the department.

- Assist unit nurse-managers as needed and requested in unit-level inservice programs.

- Knowledge and skill sessions specific to a unit.

- Problem solving clinics.

- Clinical conferences specific to a unit.

- On-the-job training for new procedures and tasks specific to unit.

<table>
<tr><td><u>Staff development department</u></td><td><u>Patient unit</u></td></tr>
<tr><td>

- Collaborate with other agency departments in programs as appropriate.
- On-the-job training for agency and department-wide procedures and tasks.

3. For Continuing Education
- Plan, organize, coordinate, implement and evaluate residency program for newly graduated nurses.
- Clinical specialty development programs.
- Nurse-manager development program
- Nurse-educator programs.

</td><td>

- Assist with clinical experience aspects of residency program for the newly graduated nurse.
- Support and reinforce on the unit new learnings of self and staff for each of the programs conducted by others for unit personnel.

</td></tr>
</table>

Whatever the division of responsibilities, careful planning and decision making is required so that there is mutual understanding about who is responsible for what. When everyone is responsible then usually no one is. Managing the educational function requires an understanding of the philosophy upon which such a function is built. As one element of the foundation for PONS, there must be a stated purpose, clearly delineated objectives and specific functions spelled out for the staff development department. The director of the department should be a nurse who can function as a facilitator, coordinator, teacher and manager. Organizationally, such a person should be in a staff rather than a line position in relation to the rest of the nursing department. As such, he or she can be viewed by the nursing staff as a valuable resource person. Thus the job requires that this director be flexible, creative and knowledgeable about current healthcare concepts, issues and trends as they relate to nursing; be able to listen to the needs and problems of others, and use confluent educational principles; and be attuned to the learning needs of both the staff development instructors and the nursing staff throughout the agency, using the results of nursing audit to help identify such current learning needs.

PATIENT EDUCATION

The level of satisfaction with patient education in most healthcare settings can be improved. Many agencies are making strenuous efforts to upgrade this vital aspect of patient care services. Patient education is more complex than it may first appear to be. What is involved is a change process, actually altering the way a person eats, exercises, sleeps, walks, bathes, uses various parts of his body, adjusts to the wearing or manipulation of a prosthesis, takes medication and modifies the habits of a lifetime. These and other adjustments may seem complex and even frightening to the patient or client. The problem is compounded by such things as the patient's values, cultural background, religion, education, life style, the influence of family and friends, past experience, superstition, misinformation, fear, and apathy.

People change themselves and their habits only when they want to or need to. Change, like motivation, is a personal thing. Change has much to do with motivation. Learning has more to do with achieving personal change than does teaching. Thus the nurse needs to be aware of what the patient is learning. Careful chronological documentation of a patient's learning progress can prove to be an invaluable source of information to all nursing staff members caring for that patient in preparation for discharge. The patient teaching flow sheet previously described in Chapter 2 is an example of one way to go about documenting the teaching objectives and learning achievements as part of a patient's progress. This flow sheet is used as part of the implementation phase of the nursing process. It is a part of the nursing plan of care and is used throughout the patient's entire care program.

The use of the patient teaching flow sheet is an example of combining the technical and human modes for the benefit of patient care. The flow sheet itself is technical mode: the form had to be designed and produced—simple enough for ease of use but complete enough for documentation purposes in connection with nursing audit. Plans had to be made for its introduction, acceptance and use as part of the medical record. The human mode aspects were uppermost in considering the form in relation to its purposeful use by the patient care team—as part of the problem-oriented nursing system, discharge planning and the patient's motivation to follow through during and after his hospitalization. Well-designed tools and systems help make possible the effective use of the human mode; they never are substitutes for it.

The Job Instruction Training (JIT) program of years past helped many persons learn how to teach job skills to new employees. The four steps of "How to Instruct" are relevant to teaching patients certain skills such as injections, dressings and other procedures they or their families will have to do at home. The following step-by-step guide for getting ready to instruct and then giving the intruction is an adaptation from the JIT program:

GET READY TO INSTRUCT

Have a Timetable
How much skill or knowledge is the learner expected to have, by what date?
Break Down the Task (or learning segment)
List important steps.
Pick out the key points. (Safety is always a key point.)
Have Everything Ready
The right equipment, materials, and supplies.
Have the Workplace Properly Arranged
Just as the learner will be expected to keep it.

HOW TO INSTRUCT

Step 1: Prepare the Learner
Put him at ease.
State the procedure (or learning segment) and find out what he already knows about it.
Get him interested in learning the procedure.
Place in correct position (if pertinent).
Step 2: Present the Procedure (or learning segment)
Tell, show, illustrate one important step at a time.
Stress each key point.
Instruct clearly, completely, and patiently, but no more than he can master.
Step 3: Try-Out Performance
Have him do the procedure (return demonstration); correct errors.
Have him explain each key point to you as he does the procedure again.
Continue until you know he knows--and can do it.
Step 4: Follow Through
Put him on his own. Designate to whom he goes for help. Document progress.
Check frequently. Encourage questions.
Taper off extra coaching and follow-up.

The true worth of what the patient and family have really learned can be identified when the label "patient" is removed and the "person" once again joins the ranks of society outside the confines of the healthcare agency. The true indicators of successful patient teaching and learning are the changes the person decides to make in life style to continue his recovery and to prevent or forestall further health problems and hospitalization.

This chapter has dealt with one of the three major responsibilities of the nurse manager, namely, that of human resources development for patients, families and staff members. This responsibility deserves equal emphasis with the responsibilities for patient care management and operational management in the day-to-day delivery of healthcare.

NOTES

1. George Isaac Brown, *Human Teaching for Human Learning* (New York: The Viking Press, Compass Books, 1972), p.3.
2. Robert Ornstein, *The Psychology of Consciousness* (San Francisco: W.H. Freeman, 1972).
3. Marilyn Ferguson, ed., "University Conference: Split-Brain Research and Education," *Brain/Mind Bulletin,* 1 (Dec. 15, 1975), p.1.
4. Virginia Gierke, "The Philosophy and Objectives of the Nursing Service Department," a report submitted in a course on Patient Care Administration at the University of Minnesota, April 30, 1976.
5. Margaret L. Pohl, *Teaching Function of the Nurse Practitioner* (DuBuque: Wm. C. Brown Co., 1968), pp. 8-13.
6. Carl Rogers, *Freedom to Learn* (Columbus: Merrill Publishing, 1969), pp. 157-164.
7. Rogers, ibid.
8. Rogers, ibid.

SUGGESTED READINGS

Books

Bloom, Benjamin. *Taxonomy of Educational Objectives. Handbook I: Cognitive Domain* (New York: David McKay, 1956).

Brown, George I. *Human Teaching for Human Learning: An Introduction to Confluent Education* (New York: Viking Press, Compass Books, 1972).

Burton, W., Kimball, R. and Wing, R. *Education for Effective Thinking* (New York: Appleton-Century-Crofts, 1960).

Cyrs, Thomas E. *You, Behavioral Objectives and Nutrition Education* (Chicago: National Dairy Council, 1973).

Dewey, John, *Experience and Education* (New York: Collier-MacMillan, 1963).

Ganong, Joan and Warren. *HELP with Innovative Teaching Techni-

ques (Chapel Hill, N.C.: W.L. Ganong Co., 1976).

Gordon, T. *Teacher Effectiveness Training* (New York: Peter H. Wyden, 1974).

Highet, Gilbert. *The Art of Teaching* (New York: Random House, Vintage Books, 1950).

Johnson, Rita B. *Humanizing Instruction or...Helping Your Students Up the Up Staircase* (Chapel Hill, N.C.: Self-Instructional Packages, 1972).

Jonas, Gerald. *Visceral Learning* (New York: Viking Press, 1973).

Krathwohl, D.R., et al. *Taxonomy of Educational Objectives, Handbook II: Affective Domain* (New York: David McKay, 1964).

Lau, J.B. *Behavior in Organizations: An Experiential Approach* (Homewood, Ill.: Richard D. Irwin, 1975).

Leonard, George. *Education and Ecstasy* (New York: Delacorte, 1968).

Mager, Robert. *Developing Attitude Toward Learning* (Belmont, Calif.: Fearon, 1968).

Mager, Robert. *Measuring Instructional Intent* (Belmont, Calif.: Fearon, 1973).

Moustakas, Clark. *Creativity and Conformity* (Princeton: Van Nostrand, Insight Books, 1968).

Ott, Herbert and Mann, John. *Ways of Growth—Approaches to Expanding Awareness* (New York: Viking Press, Compass Books, 1968).

Perls, F.S. and Hefferline, R.F. *Gestalt Therapy: Excitement and Growth in the Human Personality* (New York: Julian Press, 1951).

Pfeiffer, J.W. and Jones, J.E., eds. *A Handbook of Structural Experiences for Human Relations Training*, Vol. I and II. (Iowa City: University Associates, 1973).

Pohl, Margaret L. *Teaching Function of the Nurse Practitioner* (Dubuque: Wm. C. Brown Co., 1969).

Popiel, Elda. *Nursing and the Process of Continuing Education* (St. Louis, C.V. Mosby Co., 1973).

Powell, John. *Why Am I Afraid to Tell You Who I Am?* (Niles, Ill.: Argus Communications, 1969).

Rogers, Carl. *Freedom to Learn* (Columbus: Merrill Publishing, 1969).

Raths, L., Harmin, M. and Simon, S. *Values and Teaching* (Columbus: Charles E. Merrill Publishing Co., 1966).

Samples, Bob, and Wohlford, Bob. *Opening: A Primer for Self- Actualization* (Menlo Park, Calif: Addison-Wesley, 1975).

Schechter, Daniel. *Agenda for Continuing Education: A Challenge to Health Care Institutions* (Chicago: Hospital Research and Educational Trust, 1974).

Schrank, Jeffrey. *Teaching Human Beings* (Boston: Beacon Press,

1972).

Simon, Sidney B., Howe, Leland W., and Kirschenbaum, Howard. *Values Clarification: A Handbook of Practical Strategies for Teachers and Students* (New York: Hart Publishing Co., 1972).

Stevens, John O. *Awareness: Exploring, Experimenting, Experiencing* (Moab, Utah: Real People Press, 1971).

Sutterly, D. and Donnelly, G. *Perspectives in Human Development* (Philadelphia: J.B. Lippincott, 1973).

Thayer, L. and Beeler, K., eds. *Handbook of Affective Tools and Techniques,* mimeographed. (Ypsilanti, Mich.: E. Michigan University, 1974).

Tough, Allen. *The Adult's Learning Projects: A Fresh Approach to Theory and Practice in Adult Learning,* Research in Education Series No. 1 (Toronto: Ontario Institute for Studies in Education, 1971).

Wilhelm, Richard and Baynes, Cary, trans. *The I Ching or Book of Changes.* Bollingen Series XIX. (Princeton: Princeton University Press, 1967).

Article

Ganong, Warren L. and Joan Mary, "Good Advice: Training and Education in Health Care Organizations," *Journal of Nursing Administration,* 2 (May-June 1972), p.8.

Chapter 10
Wide-Track Careers In Nursing

Wide-Track Careers in Nursing (WTC) is defined as a viable system for providing selective career options on three main tracks in nursing—the clinical, educational, and management tracks—using agency-developed criteria for continuing education, training and the related qualifying procedures. Such a system encourages and allows nursing personnel within a single agency to grow and develop in status, responsibility and pay along the track selected and to shift from one track to another as opportunity permits.

THE RATIONALE

Earlier chapters have referred to some of the needs, problems and opportunities in connection with careers for nurses and other healthcare personnel. While much has been written and discussed about career ladders and planned job progression, specific examples of successful program applications are all too few. In fact, the requirements of the agencies which license, certify and educate healthcare occupational and professional personnel sometimes seem deliberately designed to frustrate and discourage the person who seeks upward mobility in the field of healthcare. For many persons the time and economic considerations alone—in spite of governmental and labor union financial support programs—are enough to sidetrack their motivation to undertake the prescribed qualifying routine. And for nurses, as a capstone to this escalating educational edifice, is the discovery that after a 4-year or even 5-year program leading to a bachelor's degree with the privilege of taking an examination for state licensure as a registered nurse, the coveted and hard-earned RN has no more meaning legally[1] or in being considered a nurse than does the RN earned by passing the same state board examination as a graduate of a 2-year associate-degree program or a 2 or 3-year hospital school of nursing program — the latter, at this writing, showing signs of coming back into vogue.

In addition, the observant RN soon learns through experience that many long-service LPN's and some nurse aides are performing satisfactorily a significantly high percentage (80-90%) of the tasks and procedures once the responsibility of the registered nurse. At the same time, a trend in some hospitals has been to assign broad nursing management and administrative functions to nonnurse unit managers, coordinators or assistant and associate hospital administrators. These trends over recent decades have in fact been encouraged and promoted by some nursing leaders and accepted passively by other nursing educators and practitioners. Current attempts to reassess the meaning of these trends and to evaluate their success in terms of patient care and their implications for nursing are long overdue, painful and of great concern to all nurse managers. And well they should be! Nurse managers by definition are leaders within their own agencies and are in a position to exert meaningful, assertive leadership in their professions of nursing and management. Unless you do so you have little reason to complain of the results of leadership provided by others. The proliferation of labor unions in the healthcare field provides an additional challenge and opportunity for you to demonstrate your leadership capabilities.

Other factors are at work too which influence nursing education and practice. An increasing number of master's and doctoral programs for nurses place their emphasis upon a high-skill level of clinical patient care for professional practitioners. Graduates of such programs are finding increasing opportunities as nurse practitioners in various clinical specialties in public health agencies, community centers and medical practice groups, as consultants, and as independent general nurse practitioners. One hurdle to more extensive use of such types of nurse practitioners yet to be overcome is the lack of payment for their individual services as part of third-party-payor contractual arrangements. This impediment is in the process of being resolved.

Other advanced-degree graduates are finding opportunities in hospitals as clinical specialists, nurse clinicians, primary nurses, patient care coordinators and related roles. Such well-educated clinical nurses sometimes encounter misunderstanding and lack of acceptance in the traditional hospital healthcare environment. The degree of acceptance varies with the caliber of orientation provided for the clinicians themselves and for the agency personnel for whom they are expected to become a valued resource. Much depends also upon the interpersonal skills of the individual clinicians and the particular nurse manager with whom they become associated. All too often neither party — the clinician or the nurse manager — has a clear conceptualization of the role relationships they must establish in an already complex socially layered organizational structure. With adequate planning, patience and goodwill, a successful working relationship can be achieved so that the patient benefits.

One advantage of the primary nursing concept as an alternative method for the delivery of patient care is that it usually is an adaptation of the existing nursing process within the hospital. It becomes part of a transitional participative process, realigning and expanding the roles of present nursing personnel. Carefully introduced, it offers the possibility of achieving the patient-care goals sought through the introduction of the nurse practitioner specialists, but with greater success. However, as with any innovation, success depends as much upon the process of implementation as upon the validity of the concept. And the success of the process in turn depends upon the knowledgeability and skills of the nurse manager in the three major areas of responsibility — clinical management, operational management and human resources management.

The comments of the preceding paragraph apply also to the introduction of the problem-oriented nursing system. PONS is another example of how nurses can introduce and successfully implement an innovative management technique designed to enhance patient care through a planned transitional process. PONS builds upon the existing patient care medical model; it supplements and strengthens the nursing process as presently practiced; it accepts and functions within the established organizational structure and the realities of the ongoing medical-administrative-nursing staff relationships; it places faith in the nurse-as-manager for successful implementation; it permits nurses — from whatever educational program — to practice nursing in a manner commensurate with their visions of professional nursing; and PONS helps to provide the kind of inspirational environment that encourages nursing personnel to pursue their career inclinations and goals upon the wide track of nursing opportunities.

None of the foregoing should be interpreted as an endorsement or critique per se of any particular kind of nursing. There has been a tendency during recent decades to create names to describe a variety of programmatic concepts for the delivery of nursing care. The names given to some of the popular approaches include functional nursing, team nursing, case method and primary nursing. These kinds of nursing approaches and others as well have resulted from the natural striving of nursing leaders to improve nursing's contribution to patient care within the multifaceted healthcare delivery system of our country. Problems arise, however, when enthusiastic followers and practitioners begin to espouse a particular brand name nursing method with missionary zeal and fervor. The time has come, we believe, for nurses to be able to refer to nursing in the same way that physicians refer to medicine. Nursing does not need, any more than does medicine, several brand name versions competing in this year's popularity contest. Hence our emphasis upon functions, techniques and skills rather than upon a new way of delivering patient or nursing care.

Wide-track careers in nursing must be considered in the context of one other set of facts about healthcare in this country. AHA statistics for 1973 indicated that approximately one-half (52%) of all community hospitals in this country had less than 100 beds, but these hospitals employed only 13% of all hospital personnel. All hospitals in the size category of less than 300 beds comprised 85% of all community hospitals, employing 48% of all hospital personnel in 1973. The remaining 15% of the community hospitals were over 300 beds in size, employing 52% of the personnel. However, the eleven-year trend from 1963 through 1973 showed a marked decrease in the less than 100-bed hospitals. The increase was 72% for community hospitals in the 400-499 bed range, and 88% for those with 500 or more beds. These data — and other related statistical information connected with personnel utilization, costs, career opportunities and nationwide trends in the delivery of healthcare — document the urgency of organized programs for facilitating career progress for all categories of personnel in hospitals both large and small. For nursing personnel, a wide-track careers program, as adapted to particular healthcare agencies or groups of agencies, provides an organized, effective plan for action. Here is one such application:

REAP: THE REX HOSPITAL EXAMPLE

The Rex Employee Advancement Program or REAP is the name given to the wide-track careers program as it was implemented by the nursing department of Rex Hospital in Raleigh, N.C. This program proved to be an undertaking of major proportions. It was approved by Joseph E. Barnes, Director of Rex Hospital, and initiated after the nursing department had experienced a period of self-development and organizational renewal under the leadership of Sarah Hitchcock, Director of Nursing, in a most favorable professional environment for innovation. Organizational changes had included expanding to all patient care units the patient care coordinator concept which had been introduced earlier as a pilot project on one of the large patient care units. Not long thereafter the hospital school of nursing was phased out as another aspect of financial and program planning.

The initial planning and implementation efforts for REAP were carried out by the patient care coordinators and other staff personnel including the inservice education director and the staffing coordinator. This hard-working group produced the initial drafts of the lengthy task lists for the different job categories which serve as helpful criteria for the different job levels. These lists were later reviewed and refined by head nurses and other nursing staff representatives from the different units.

Another vital phase of the project was the writing of performance descriptions for all positions in the nursing department. These follow the format used in other chapters of this book (see Chapters 1 and 4). They replaced the existing job descriptions and serve not only to define the major responsibilities for the persons in each job category, but also provide the basis for results-oriented performance evaluation.

The next section of this chapter presents the description of REAP as developed by the nursing department for its staff members, the membership and objectives of the REAP committee, policy statements covering the program, and a sampling of the performance descriptions and task lists being used. As with any worthwhile program, continuing maintenance and updating is required. The REAP Committee meets as necessary to revise and refine important elements of the total plan. One such element is the criteria used for identifying the job levels in each position category and for evaluating the readiness of a person for promotion from one job level to another and from one position category to another. Work is being done to augment the task lists with criteria relating more directly to skill in using the nursing process and related patient care programs.

REX HOSPITAL NURSING DEPARTMENT

Rex Employee Advancement Program

The Rex Employee Advancement Program (REAP) was developed within Nursing Service to maintain and improve the caliber of patient care, to increase growth and income opportunities for Nursing Service personnel and to achieve these goals while decreasing the relative rate of operating expenses. It was felt that such a program should be implemented to assist in meeting the present and future staffing needs in the Nursing Department at Rex Hospital. The following factors have the potential for making these needs more acute:

1. The closing of diploma Schools of Nursing in North Carolina, including our own Rex Hospital School of Nursing, will greatly decrease the resources for recruitment.
2. The trend toward increased utilization of LPNs and graduates of Associate Degree programs will require that the employer provide for intensive and extensive orientation as well as continuing education.
3. The turnover rate among the Nursing Assistants is creating a cost factor that must be dealt with in terms of dollars and cents as well as the amount of Inservice Education time that must be spent in training. This time could be better utilized in the development of personnel already on the staff.

People have varied ideas of career planning and development. This is as it should be, since the subject is a matter of such personal concern. Yet it is also a matter of vital organization concern, since the survival and well-being of Rex Hospital is dependent upon those who build their careers here. Thus, mutually understood concepts, assumptions, and procedures which best achieve the goals of all individuals and the organization are needed. A number of such concepts and considerations are are set forth below:

1. People are one of the most important assets at Rex Hospital. This is a fundamental belief that forms the foundation for Rex's administrative philosophy and for its personnel policies and procedures.
2. "Career" means a person's lifework, profession, occupation. As the term "Career" is used here, it means also "one's advancement or achievement in a particular vocation." Some persons may prefer the broader definition of "one's progress through life."
3. Each person's career is of mutual concern to him and to Rex Hospital. Both parties are making a substantial and often critical investment in the employment contract. Both have a right to expect some advantage, gain and benefit from such employment. Both parties need to work actively and cooperatively together toward such benefit. Rex Hospital provides these types of self-development and personal growth opportunities which permit every person to advance as far as he is able.

4. Responsibility for an individual's career rests with the individual alone. This is a simple fact. As much as the hospital may wish to help with the progress of an employee only he can be responsible for himself. He is responsible for what happens in his progress through life and occupation. As working plans are made, it is important to consider not only what one thinks he may *want* to do, but also what one *can* do (assets and liabilities), and what one *likes* to do.

5. Each employee's supervisor has a responsibility to assist him in his work and career development. Supervisors know that this is a key responsibility. They know that they help themselves when they help their people with their jobs and growth. They can suggest other sources of help when they feel it is needed and can be useful. Some of these sources are within the hospital. Others are outside the hospital, and some are within the employee himself.

6. The Rex Hospital concept of a statisfactory career accommodates everything from one with *no* job changes to one with many changes and promotions. Some persons are quite happy to do a good job of what they are already doing, and do not seek promotion. Others want to feel that they can move along into more complicated clinical jobs, or take on administrative responsibilities. Rex Hospital Employee Advancement Program for Nursing Service personnel makes room for many types of career success definitions within the framework of "advancement or achievement in a particular vocation." Together, these varied career-successes contribute to keeping Rex Hospital "Tops in Patient Care" and "A Good Place to Work."

7. The Rex Hospital Employee Advancement Program offers many opportunities for job satisfaction and for growth if desired.

- on present job
- within technical specialty
- within nursing administration
- into other hospital functions
- outward to other health care agencies

Rex Hospital Employee Advancement Program has the following features and benefits:

1. Identifies for *all* nursing service employees the pathways to earned promotions and merited increases in pay.

2. Provides both clinical and managerial promotional channels for qualified personnel beyond the present RN practitioner level.

3. Establishes standards of performance and a performance review plan for all job levels.
4. Provides additional promotional steps within specific job categories (NA, RN, LPN, WS).
5. Permits merit pay increases within job categories as promotions are earned from one step to another, based upon ability to satisfactorily perform additional tasks.
6. Assures qualified persons of Nursing Service positions.
7. Permits staffing each unit with the minimum number of qualified personnel with the resultant savings in wage costs.
8. Requires that persons who qualify for higher job levels be able to perform all tasks identified for lower-paid job levels and to actually perform those tasks when staffing emergencies occur.

At present there are approximately twenty levels for Nursing Service personnel. Each level is defined with established criteria and performance descriptions. These performance descriptions are utilized in the evaluation of Nursing Service personnel. Attached to each job description is a Task List which indicates the nursing tasks that can be performed by personnel at each level.

The REAP Committee

Primary Objective

To contribute to the improvement and maintenance of high caliber patient care by providing and evaluating increasing growth opportunities for all Nursing Service personnel.

Contributory Objectives

1. To assist in keeping the Rex Hospital Employee Advancement Program for nursing personnel up-to-date.
2. To evaluate recommendations received regarding the REAP Program.
3. To serve as a liaison between all nursing personnel and the committee.

Membership

Composed of at least one representative for each level of nursing personnel with each nursing unit being represented. Members serve a one year term, from January to January.

Statement of Policy (1)

Nursing Units Affected: All Units
Effective: July 29, 1974, the following Rex Hospital Employee Advancement Program policies will be activated:

1. The classification of Nursing Service personnel at Rex Hospital shall be determined in accordance with the criteria established in the Rex Hospital Employee Advancement Program. (It is expected that these employees will move through the classifications at different rates depending on such factors as academic preparation, previous experience, ability to apply knowledge, and motivation.)

2. The advancement of Nursing Service personnel from level to level will be determined by a meritorious performance evaluation with a subsequent recommendation from the Head Nurse and Patient Care Coordinator for the employee to begin preparation for the next level. When the basic criteria as established for that particular level in the Rex Hospital Employee Advancement Program has been attained, he or she is eligible for advancement with the appropriate salary adjustment being made.

Exceptions to the above:

A. The practical nurse will advance to the LPN I level when licensure is obtained.

B. The graduate professional nurse will advance to the RN I level when licensure is obtained.

C. There shall be no ninety day waiting period for the RN I and LPN I to be recommended by the Head Nurse and Patient Care Coordinator to begin preparation for the levels of RN II and LPN II.

D. The practical nurse may take the Medication Qualifying Examination before obtaining licensure; however, only after becoming licensed, may he or she pursue becoming certified in medication administration or participation in the Inservice Medication Course.

E. The graduate professional nurse may attend the certification programs offered through Inservice Education; however, supervision for certification in these procedures cannot be initiated until licensure is obtained.

3. The actual level advancement will occur only at the time a position for that specific level becomes available.

4. All Nursing Service employees whose qualifications fulfill the established requirements for each level as specified in the Rex Hospital Employee Advancement Program should become eligible for positions of advancement within the Nursing Service Department. In order to insure every applicant the considerations that are due him/her, the following procedure will be followed.

A. Vacant positions for levels will be announced. A time limit will be established for receiving applications when appropriate.

B. Eligible applicants should submit a Special Request Form to the Director of Nursing stating his or her qualifications and reasons for seeking the position.

C. The applicant's form of request in addition to his or her evaluations and recommendations by the Head Nurse and Patient Care Coordinator will be reviewed by the Director of Nursing and Patient Care Coordinator from the unit with the existing vacancy.

D. The employee to fill the position will be selected with priority given to the one who has been prepared for the longest period of time for that specific level and whose qualifications are adequate for the position.

E. Priority for filling positions that would allow for level advancement will be given to the existing Nursing Service personnel before a new employee is hired for the position.

5. If an employee does not merit advancement through variable performance or lack of motivation, the preexisting classification status and the salary scale shall be maintained. If necessary, the employee may be reclassified to the level which best describes his or her current performance with the necessary salary adjustment being made.

6. The Programs stipulated as being necessary for level advancement in the Rex Hospital Employee Advancement Program shall be offered by Rex Hospital through the Inservice Education Department or through other health-related agencies. Programs provided by other agencies must be evaluated and recommended by the Inservice Education Department as meeting the pre-preparational needs of that specific level.

7. Any educational program attended prior to employment at Rex Hospital that appears similar in content to the program required by the criteria for a particular level must be deemed comparable by the Rex Hospital Inservice Education Department before credit will be granted.

8. The graduate professional nurse will be hired at Rex Hospital at the RN I salary scale; however, he or she shall be classified as a graduate nurse performing only those tasks assigned to the graduate nurse level as specified by the Rex Hospital Employee Advancement Program.

9. The graduate professional nurse at Rex Hospital will be allowed one year from the date the first State Board Examination is offered after his or her graduation to successfully obtain his or her licensure. If at the end of this period of time, he or she has not successfully obtained licensure, he or she shall be reclassified into the LPN III salary scale; however, his or her level classification shall remain that of a graduate nurse and he or she shall continue ot perform only those tasks specified for the graduate nurse level by the Rex Hospital Employee Advancement Program. If no position for this level employee exists on the unit assigned, a transfer to a unit with a vacancy for this level may be necessary.

10. The graduate professional nurse who has been unsuccessful in obtaining his or her licensure prior to applying for a position at Rex Hospital shall be hired at the LPN III salary scale if more than one year from the date the first State Board Examination was offered after his or her graduation has elapsed. However, he or she shall be classified in the graduate nurse performance level and shall be assigned only those tasks specified for the graduate nurse level by the Rex Hospital Employee Advancement Program.

11. The graduate practical nurse will be hired at Rex Hospital at the LPN I salary scale; however, he or she shall be classified as a practical nurse performing only those tasks assigned to the practical nurse level as specified by the Rex Hospital Employee Advancement Program.

12. The graduate practical nurse at Rex Hospital will be allowed one year from the date the first State Board Examination is offered after his or her graduation to successfully obtain his or her licensure. If at the end of this period of time, he or she has not successfully obtained licensure, he or she shall be reclassified into the NA III salary scale; however, his or her level classification shall remain that of a practical nurse and he or she shall continue to perform only those tasks specified for the practical nurse level by the Rex Hospital Employee Advancement Program. If no position for this level employee exists on the unit assigned a transfer to a unit with a vacancy for this level may be necessary.

13. The graduate practical nurse who has been unsuccessful in obtaining his or her licensure prior to applying for a position at Rex

Hospital shall be hired at the NA III salary scale if more than one year from the date the first State Board Examination was offered after his or her graduation has elapsed. However, he or she shall be classified in the practical nurse performance level and shall be assigned only those tasks specified for the practical nurse level by the Rex Hospital Employee Advancement Program.

14. Exceptions to the criteria established for the individual levels of Nursing Service personnel by the Rex Hospital Employee Advancement Program may be granted by the Director of Nursing based upon the written recommendation of the Patient Care Coordinator who has evaluated the employee's knowledge and skills and previous experience.

15. A new employee whose education and previous experience based upon acceptable references meet the established criteria for a level with the exception of specific required certification programs may be hired into the level and be allowed ninety days to become certified in all the procedures. If at the end of ninety days, certification has not been attained he or she shall be reclassified into the appropriate level with the necessary salary adjustment being made.

16. A new employee may be hired into the level of Nursing Service established by the Rex Hospital Employee Advancement Program as is indicated by his or her education and previous experience based upon acceptable references for a ninety day period of evaluation. At the end of this time, a written evaluation will be done and if he or she is functioning unsatisfactorily for that level, a reclassification in level may be necessary with the appropriate salary adjustment being made.

Origin of Policies: Department of Nursing
Originated: July 23, 1974
Revised: December 22, 1975

Signed: (Director of Nursing, Assistant Director of Nursing, Director of Rex Hospital)

Statement of Policy (2)

Nursing Units Affected: All Units
Effective July 9, 1975, the following policy will be activated regarding check-off of nursing tasks designed for each level in the Rex Employee Advancement Program:
A satisfactory check-off of all nursing tasks designated as core tasks on the REAP Nursing Activities Task List must be accomplished

within ninety days of the completion of an Inservice Education class offered as preparation for a higher level. The action taken upon failure to accomplish this check-off will be at the discretion of the Patient Care Coordinator. Exceptions may be granted only upon the recommendation of the Patient Care Coordinator. Those other tasks designated as occuring infrequently or only in specialty nursing areas are to be checked-off as they occur.

A satisfactory check-off is required on those tasks designated as occuring in specialty nursing areas only for nursing personnel assigned to those areas.

Nursing Service personnel who transfer from a medical-surgical area to a specialty area or from a specialty area to a medical-surgical area will be granted a 90-day evaluation period at the time of their transfer. This will allow ample time for the check-off of necessary tasks and for an evaluation of performance in that area to be done by the Head Nurse and/or Patient Care Coordinator.

Origin of Policy: Patient Care Coordinators
                  Systems and Planning
                  Inservice Education
Originated: July 1, 1975

Signed: (Director of Nursing, Coordinator of Inservice Education, Director of Rex Hospital)

IN CONCLUSION

The concept of wide-track careers reaches beyond the confines of a single healthcare agency. Career ladders must necessarily allow the nurse to move freely and to advance in a variety of work settings along the track or tracks available—clinical, education, or management. The number and variety of such growth and career opportunities continue to expand, and include the option of independent practice. The use of the wide-track careers concept, by whatever name, is essential to provide suitable opportunities for motivated nurses to prepare themselves for advancement in responsibility, status and remuneration.

We look upon nurses, especially nurse managers, as people with unique opportunities to live full and meaningful lives through their impact upon the lives of others. Our attempt in this book has been to share with you a variety of beliefs, techniques and skills which will enrich your own life and work through your helping relationships with patients, families, coworkers, and professional and community groups. No one can force you to use the contents of this book or of any other source of guidance. Only you can motivate you. By the same token, no one can prevent you from growing; from understanding the five basic human needs and how to utilize that knowledge; or from becoming skilled as a nurse manager. You, The Nurse, are one of our most valued national resources — a resource that becomes enriched rather than depleted through use.

NOTES

1. This situation may change by 1985, in at least one state, if the New York State Nurses' Association's "85 Resolution" becomes law. A legislative bill calls for a mandatory baccalaureate degree for nurse licensure. See *RN Magazine*, May 1976, p. 10. *Hospital Week* for May 28, 1976, reports that the AHA Board of trustees voted to oppose "with full vigor" legislative efforts under way in several states to limit by 1985 registered nurse licensure to graduates of baccalaureate programs. Also see John A. Wilkinson, "Hospital Schools of Nursing: Profits Counterpoise Costs," *Hospitals*, 50 (April 16, 1976), p. 95-98.

SUGGESTED READINGS

Books

American Hospital Association. *Career Mobility: A Guide for Program Planning in Health Occupations* (Chicago: AHA, 1971).
Lysaught, J.P., ed. *Action in Nursing: Progress in Professional Purpose* (New York: McGraw-Hill, 1974).

Articles

Anderson, Margaret Ives, and Denyes, Mary Jean, "A Ladder for Clinical Advancement in Nursing Practice, Implementation," *Journal of Nursing Administration*, 5 (February 1975), pp. 16-22.
Colavecchio, Ruth; Tescher, Barbara; and Scalzi, Cynthia, "A Clinical Ladder for Nursing Practice," *Nursing Digest*, 3 (January- February 1975), pp. 5-9.
McClure, Margaret L., "Entry into Professional Practice: The New York Proposal," *Journal of Nursing Administration*, 6 (June 1976), pp. 12-17.

Reichow, Ronald and Scott, Robert, "Study Compares Graduates of Two-, Three-, and Four-Year Programs," *Hospitals*, 50 (July 16, 1976), pp. 95-100.

Appendix A

General Performance Responsibilities
of Administrative and
Management Personnel

PURPOSE: Deliver the required health care services consistent with the charter, philosophy, and objectives of your agency.

MAJOR PERFORMANCE
RESPONSIBILITIES:

PERFORMANCE IS SATISFACTORY
WHEN:

I. To Administrator or Manager

A. Organizational
  1. Function within the general policies, stated beliefs and philosophy of Community General Hospital.

The hospital is represented to people within and without the organization with a general feeling of support and implementation of these policies and beliefs through both written and oral expression.

  2. Maintain clear lines of authority and responsibility.

Up-to-date department policies and performance descriptions are maintained.

  3. Obtain your own manager's approval of departmental policies and organizational plans.

Approval is obtained before establishing such policies or plans.

B. Operational
  1. Prepare and administer departmental budget.

Department is operated within approved budgets; reasonable cost standards are developed and maintained; cost and budgets are periodically reviewed.

  2. Perform or supervise record-keeping.

Records are maintained currently, are understandable to all personnel who use them, and meet legal or other requirements.

MAJOR PERFORMANCE
RESPONSIBILITIES:

PERFORMANCE IS SATISFACTORY
WHEN:

3. Establish specific goals and objectives for the department.

Such goals are in writing and include target dates for completion; and are prepared with the help of department personnel.

4. Plan, schedule and coordinate the day-to-day work activities.

The necessary work is accomplished effectively.

C. <u>Communications</u>
1. Keep your manager informed of current departmental activities, plans and developments through both oral and written reports.

Administration is informed of departmental objectives and plans, status of work and programs, personnel matters and performance of subordinates as appropriate; regular and special reports are accurate, complete, and submitted on time. "Never let your boss be surprised!"

2. Answer correspondence.

Correspondence is acted upon within 24 hours.

D. <u>Developmental</u>
1. Keep abreast of latest developments affecting your area of responsibility; keep own supervisor informed of such developments.

Your own manager is kept informed of new developments; recommendations are made as to how methods, procedures and quality may be improved through these developments.

2. Participate in research and experimental projects that are desirable and appropriate for the hospital.

Research and experimental projects improve patient care and services, employee relations, and the public or professional image of the hospital.

3. Plan and implement programs that improve the hospital's service to the community.

Provide written proposals for your manager's approval that:
(a) identify needs and issues concerning the department;
(b) structure issues in terms of alternative courses of action and cost factors.

II. To Department Personnel

A. <u>Operational</u>
1. Maintain an optimum staff of qualified personnel.

There are enough people to get the work done well, but no more than necessary. Those hired have the basic requirements to become productive workers.

MAJOR PERFORMANCE RESPONSIBILITIES:	PERFORMANCE IS SATISFACTORY WHEN:
2. Carry out the wage and salary administration program conscientiously.	Wage and salary increases are recommended as soon as justified. Dissatisfactions with pay are minimal.
3. Conduct personnel activities in accordance with hospital personnel programs and policies.	Policies and procedures are carried out effectively; necessary exceptions receive approval.
4. Maintain equipment in good operating condition.	Regular monthly inspections are conducted; needed repairs are effected; units are replaced when repairing would be inadequate.
5. Maintain adequate quality and quantity of materials and supplies.	No work interruptions occur because of "out-of-stock items."
6. Build a departmental environment which encourages maximum motivation of employees.	Employees show self-motivation rather than having to be pushed to get the work done.
7. Develop improved systems and procedures.	Evidence exists that these lead to easier ways of doing the work, to improved performance results, and minimum cost.

B. <u>Training and Safety</u>

1. Supervise training and orientation of subordinates.	Subordinates to be trained have been identified; types of experiences and training needed has been planned; subordinates are actively obtaining such experience or training; periodic evaluation is made of subordinates' progress; there is evidence of development of subordinates in terms of their results.
2. Supervise compliance of personnel with safety regulations and sanitation requirements.	Accidents do not occur to personnel or equipment because of violations of these regulations; the area is clean and orderly at all times; formal inspections disclose no violation of regulations.
3. Supervise training of personnel to cope with emergency situations such as fire, disaster, etc.	Personnel attend orientation and Fire & Safety Training Programs as scheduled; personnel are kept informed of procedures or developments that affect their performance in emergency situations.

MAJOR PERFORMANCE RESPONSIBILITIES:	PERFORMANCE IS SATISFACTORY WHEN:
C. Communications	
1. Keep subordinates informed of current changes that affect them.	Subordinates are informed promptly of hospital and departmental plans, policies, procedures, etc., that affect their work, welfare and morale.
2. Maintain an effective upward flow of information.	Feelings, opinions and attitudes of employees are sought, obtained and used as a basis for management action.
3. Resolve personnel problems.	Listening and counselling results in improved situation.
D. Developmental	
1. Evaluate employee performance.	Every employee "knows where he stands" at all times. Formal appraisals are carried out as scheduled.
2. Encourage full self-development of all employees.	Ongoing training is planned and conducted to improve the quality of employee performance; there is evidence of improvement in work results. Employees are advanced to higher-rated jobs as they qualify for existing openings.
3. Stimulate employee participation in planning for the immediate and long-range future.	Plans are made with the assistance of subordinates whenever possible; subordinates participate, within reason, in the setting of objectives.

III.   To Other Departments

MAJOR PERFORMANCE RESPONSIBILITIES:	PERFORMANCE IS SATISFACTORY WHEN:
A. Operational	
1. Work cooperatively with other departments to accomplish hospital objectives.	Evidence exists that there are successful communications and harmonious working relationships among departments.
B. Communications	
1. Participate in hospital meetings.	Attendance is regular and participation is meaningful.
C. Developmental	
1. Provide instruction for other departments as required.	Appropriate instruction is provided as scheduled.

MAJOR PERFORMANCE RESPONSIBILITIES:	PERFORMANCE IS SATISFACTORY WHEN:

IV. To Other Organizations

A. <u>Communications</u>
1. Participate in activities of outside organizations to provide information on hospital activities and plans, explain the hospital's role and position in the health care field and in the community, promote the public image of the hospital; and to obtain for the benefit of the hospital such information and opinions as may be useful in guiding management action.

Suitable participation is provided to outside agencies as requested, or as sought; adequate feedback is provided and evaluated in time to be of value in influencing administrative planning and action.

2. Prepare reports as requested by federal, state, community agencies, hospital associations, etc.

Reports are accurate, complete and are submitted on time; duplicate copies are retained for hospital records.

B. <u>Developmental</u>
1. Participate in professional and technical society meetings pertinent to own areas of special interest.

Attendance and participation is meaningful.

Appendix B

Summary Worksheet
Our Principles of Nursing Practice

SUMMARY WORKSHEET
OUR PRINCIPLES OF NURSING PRACTICE

NAME ________________________________   AGENCY ______________________________

DEPT. or UNIT ___________________   DATE ____________________________

As developed by: ____

OUR PHILOSOPHY

OUR GOALS

OUR CURRENT PATIENT CARE OBJECTIVES

DEFINITIONS FOR OUR UNIT

FUNCTIONS of OUR NURSING STAFF MEMBERS

OUR EDUCATION AND RESEARCH NEEDS

(Use additional pages as necessary)

Appendix C

Management by Objectives

An Instructional Model for Helping Others to
Learn to Write Objectives

Advance Preparation: Have available examples of well written objectives that include the components and which are pertinent for your group and type of organization.

Step # 1: Introduce written objectives in the context of the philosophy and goals of your organization. (Refer to Section 1 of HELP with Management by Objectives.) Use pertinent local examples of available statements of philosophy and goals.

Step # 2: Explain briefly how written objectives help to focus attention on worthwhile projects; assist in setting priorities for action; and help in scheduling the necessary time and money.

Step # 3: Write on the blackboard a specific statement of an objective that includes all or most of the components. Discuss briefly the meaning of this objective.

Step # 4: Write on the board, "Components of a written objective." List three components. (See Section 2 of HELP study guide.)

     1. WHAT will be done (*includes* action verb)
     2. HOW MUCH/HOW WELL
     3. WHEN (Target date)

Step # 5:   Subdivide the group into pairs. Ask each pair working together to identify the components of the specific objective as written on the blackboard. Allow the group to work together in pairs, giving such help to each pair as may be necessary to assist them in identifying the action verb, what will be done, how well, how much, and how soon.

(Note: A second example of another objective may be used to repeat this Step #5. See example at end of steps.)

Step # 6:   Summarize for the group as follows: "Each written objective must have three main components as identified. In addition, the objective may include *who* will do the what *where*, and at what *cost*." Write these items on the board.

Step # 7:   Ask the group to just sit and look at the board to "drink in" these components. Then have the group members close their eyes, while the leader erases what is on the blackboard.

Step # 8:   Ask the group to write down on a blank sheet of paper exactly what they remember from the board information.

Step # 9:   As the first and second persons look up from their sheets giving an indication that they have completed the assigned task, ask them to come forward and have each reproduce on the blackboard what they have on their written sheets.

Step #10:   Ask the rest of the group to make additions and corrections to what has been written on the blackboard.

Step #11:   Erase the blackboard.

Step #12:   Ask the group members to turn over their sheets and perform the same task of reproducing what was on the blackboard the second time.

Step #13:   Break up the group into pairs again and ask one member of each pair to explain to the other member what are the components of a written objective.

Step #14:   Ask each group member to use the specific objective as written on the board and mark over the specific words which are active verb, what will be done, how much, how well, how soon. They may also mark if it is indicated who and where.

Step #15:   Ask the whole group to give verbally, one more time, the components of a written objective.

Step #16:   Ask group to break up into triads. Each person is then to write a specific objective for himself based upon some area of real concern to him in his work situation.

Step #17:   If some of the participants finish writing an objective before the rest of the group, ask those persons to write a second objective to keep them occupied and to avoid discussion while the rest are finishing.

Step #18:   Ask members of each triad to exchange their written objectives so that each person is working with somebody else's written statement, and goes through the process of inspecting and correcting it to conform with the components checklist. Each person then receives his own written statement back and discussion ensues regarding the correct statements.

Step #19:   The groups then reform into dyads, one person to be the boss and the other the subordinate. Each member of the dyad takes his turn at presenting his written statement to "his boss" and goes through the process of attempting to develop the written statement into a mutually-developed and agreed-upon statement of objectives to which both can subscribe.

Step #20:   Entire group discusses what they have learned from the prior experience. "I learned that there is a cost attached to objectives."

Step #21:   Group is asked to discuss how they now feel about
             writing objectives.

Step #22:   Group members are asked to close their eyes and think
             about what they are now aware of.

Note:
Here is an example of a second objective that may be
used in Step #5. "Plan the allocation and scheduling of
the nursing staff so that patient needs are met at all
times on all shifts without varying more than 5 percent
from the allocated number of nursing man-hours."
Ask group members to identify again the components in
this objective, and to write-in above the words the
particular components. (This additional exercise may
help to emphasize the fact that for some objectives
the *how much* is just as important as the *how well*.)

Appendix D

285

Sample Performance Descriptions

GUIDELINES AND WORKSHEET FOR PREPARING YOUR OWN PERFORMANCE DESCRIPTION

I. Consider your own performance responsibilities. What do you do, for whom? In the space below, list four of the persons (or groups of people) for whom you have to do something. Then list two things you have to do for each as part of your performance requirements.

Persons (or Groups of People)	What I Do For Them
1.	a.
	b.
2.	a.
	b.
3.	a.
	b.
4.	a.
	b.

II. Now select one of the things you do for someone (as listed in the right hand column of Step I) which you think is easiest to measure. How do you know when you have performed <u>satisfactorily</u>? When you have decided upon your answer, complete the following sentence:

My performance for item # ___ (from Step I) is satisfactory when

____

____

____

____

III.   Take the worksheet to your own manager. Show what you have
       written for Steps I and II. Ask your boss, "Do you agree
       with what I wrote down?" Discuss and modify as necessary
       to reach agreement.

       If you are prepared to do so, show your "measures of satis-
       factory performance" for another one or two things you do
       for someone else (your "performance responsibilities").
       Discuss, and reach agreement.

       Then soon after having had your discussion with your boss,
       write below your reactions as you recall them. What were
       your feelings during the discussion? What are your feelings
       now? How might this experience influence your use of per-
       formance descriptions with your staff members?

IV.   Follow through. What you do next is up to you, influenced
       by the reactions of your boss and your own feelings. Out-
       line below your follow-through plan of action.

SELF-EVALUATION OF PERFORMANCE

NAME: ____DATE:___________________________

TITLE: ____

DEPARTMENT: ___________________________________REPORTS TO: _____________________________

PURPOSE OF YOUR WORK: (In your own words, tell the reasons for what you do.)

PERFORMANCE RESPONSIBILITIES: (In your own words, how well do you perform each
                      responsibility? Include examples of results.

A. To Patients

B. To Medical Staff

C. To Your Own Manager (supervisor)

D. To Department Personnel

E. To Committees

F. To Personnel of Other Departments (or other organizations)

G. To Self

Note: Use Additional sheets as necessary. When completed, return the sheet(s) to
       your nurse manager (or supervisor).

COMMUNITY GENERAL HOSPITAL
PERFORMANCE DESCRIPTION

TITLE: <u>R N   II</u>   DEPARTMENT: <u>Nursing Service</u>

SUPERVISES: LPN's, Nursing Assistants, Orderlies, Technicians,
Ward Clerks, Unit Service Aides

PURPOSE: To assess, plan and give nursing care at RN II level with a
minimum of assistance. Functions as a team leader or may
assume charge duties when adequately prepared.

MAJOR PERFORMANCE RESPONSIBILITIES: PERFORMANCE IS SATISFACTORY WHEN:

A. *To Patients*
1. Assist in formulating and carrying out patient care plans.
2. Evaluate care given to patients.
3. Assess the needs of the patient.
4. Act as liaison between patients, physician and family.
5. Give direct patient care as needed.
6. Performs nursing activities as assigned for RN II on Nursing Activities Task List.

1. Effective plan of care is implemented.
2. Care meets established criteria for quality and amount.
3. Needs are identified through skillful interviewing and observation, and are recorded.
4. Patient and family understand and carry out physician's directions.
5. Objectives of care plan are met.
6. These activities are carried out safely, correctly and economically.

B. *To Medical Staff*
1. Carry out physician's orders.
2. Ask for clarification of physician's orders as necessary.
3. Inform physician of changes in patient's condition.
4. Make rounds with Physician.

1. Orders are implemented with no mistakes.
2. Orders are clearly understood.
3. Information is accurately recorded and relayed.
4. Rounds assist in formulating patient care plans and provide in-depth comprehension of patient's condition.

C. *To Own Nurse Manager*
1. Report on and off duty as assigned.
2. Keep up-to-date in nursing procedures.
3. Conduct and participate in team conferences.
4. Communicate appropriate information.
5. Make out patient-care assignment.

1. Established schedule is met.
2. Competence in performing procedures is demonstrated.
3. Greater understanding of patient's condition is achieved by team members.
4. Necessary communications are passed on. (Never let your boss be surprised.)
5. Skills of team members are recognized and utilized.

MAJOR PERFORMANCE RESPONSIBILITIES:

PERFORMANCE IS SATISFACTORY WHEN:

D. *To Unit Personnel*
1. Maintain harmonious relationship with other team members.
2. Participate in unit teaching and orienting as needed.

3. Encourage proper technique and procedures.
4. Function effectively as a professional team member.

1. Own efforts contribute patient-care team work.
2. Patient care team works effectively with favorable response to instruction.
3. Safe nursing care is rendered.

4. Own performance sets desired example and facilitates team work.

E. *To Committees*
1. Actively participates in assigned committee work.
2. Attend regular meetings of appropriate unit of Nursing Service Personnel Organization.

1. Committee objectives are met.

2. Active participation is evident and there is a feeling of satisfaction with the Unit meetings.

F. *To Other Departments*
1. Carry out interdepartmental assignments and communications.

1. Positive feedback is obtained.

G. *To Other Organizations*
1. Participates in appropriate professional nursing and community organizations.

1. Such activity aids in meeting personal and hospital goals.

H. *To Self*
1. Maintain sense of personal satisfaction.
2. Participate in continuing education programs.

1. Personal goals are met as related to job performance.
2. Progress is made in preparation for promotion, and in updating job knowledge and skills.

Qualifications

1. Graduate of Accredited School of Nursing.

2. Current State Registration   (or in process of licensing).

3. Certification of those procedures required for R.N. II; certification for special procedures.

4. Completion of the Community General Hospital orientation program within thirty days of employment.

PERFORMANCE DESCRIPTION WORKSHEET

NAME: _______________________________________ DEPT: _______________________

JOB TITLE: _________________________________ DATE: _______________________

Name of your supervisor: ____

Name of your department head: ____

Names and titles of persons you supervise (if you are a supervisor or manager):

INSTRUCTIONS: You can help prepare an up-to-date Performance Description of what you do in your work. Please be as complete as possible. Do not be bashful; list everything you think is part of your job. If you need more space, use additional sheets.

---

1. The purpose of my work is ____

2. For whom are you doing your work? _____________________________________

3. How do you know whether or not you are performing your work satisfactorily? _____________

4. List anything you are doing which you think should not be part of your work: __________

5. List anything you are not doing which you think should be part of your work: __________

6. Who taught you your work? ____

7. When you started on your present job, how long did it take you to learn to do the work satisfactorily? ____

8. COMMENTS AND SUGGESTIONS: Add anything else that will help your work and how you feel about it. (Use additional sheets if you need more space): ______________

Appendix E

Bad Judgment Test

STORY A

Instructions

First, read the story. Assume that all the information presented is accurate. No need to memorize, though. You can refer back whenever you wish.

Next, read the statements. "T" means that the statement is definitely true on the basis of the information in the story. "F" means that it is definitely false. "?" what you cannot be certain of on the basis of the information in the story. If any part of a statement is doubtful, use the "?".

Circle your answer to each statement in turn. Do not go back to change any answer later. This would distort your results.

THE STORY

As you step onto your front porch from your living room you observe a delivery truck approaching along the street. You also see that your next-door neighbor is backing her car from her garage into the street in the path of the approaching truck. You see the truck swerve, climb over the curbing and come to a stop against a tree which crumples one of its front fenders.

Statements About the Story

1. Your next-door neighbor was backing her car into the street in the path of an approaching truck.   T   F   ?

2. The delivery truck was traveling at a reasonable speed.   T   F   ?

293

3. The only damage resulting from the incident was to the truck's fender.   T   F   ?

4. You saw the truck swerve and climb over the curbing.   T   F   ?

5. Your neighbor across the street was backing her car out of the garage.   T   F   ?

6. The truck suffered no damage.   T   F   ?

7. You saw the truck approaching as you stepped onto your front porch from your living room.   T   F   ?

8. The man who drove the delivery truck swerved and ran his truck up over a curbing.   T   F   ?

9. The delivery truck driver swerved in order to miss a child playing in the street.   T   F   ?

STORY B

Instructions

First, read the story. Assume that all the information presented is accurate. No need to memorize, though. You can refer back whenever you wish.

Next, read the statements. "T" means that the statement is definitely true on the basis of the information in the story. "F" means that it is definitely false. "?" what you cannot be certain of on the basis of the information in the story. If any part of a statement is doubtful, mark it "?".

Answer each statement in turn. Do not go back to change any answer later. This would distort your results.

THE STORY

John and Betty Smith are awakened in the middle of the night by a noise coming from the direction of their living room. Smith investigates and finds that the door opening into the garden, which he thought he had locked before going to bed, is standing wide open. Books and papers are scattered all over the floor, around the desk in one corner of the room.

Statements About the Story

1. Mrs. Smith was awakened in the middle of the night.   T   F   ?

2. Smith locked the door from his living room to his garden before going to bed.   T   F   ?

3. The books and papers were scattered between the time Mr. Smith went to bed and the time he was awakened.   T   F   ?

4. Smith found that the door opening onto the garden was shut.   T   F   ?

5. Mr. Smith did not lock the garden door.   T   F   ?

6. John Smith was not awakened by a noise.   T   F   ?

7. Nothing was missing from the room.   T   F   ?

8. Mrs. Smith was sleeping when she and Mr. Smith were awakened.   T   F   ?

9. While a burglar was the first thing Smith thought of when he was awakened, the story does not really make clear that there was a burglar present.   T   F   ?

10. Mr. and Mrs. Smith were awakened in the middle of the night by a noise.   T   F   ?

11. The noise did not come from their garden.   T   F   ?

12. Smith saw no burglar in the living room.   T   F   ?

Answers are on page 296.

These two test stories were developed by, and printed with the permission of, Dr. William V. Haney, Northwestern University School of Business.

ANSWERS TO THE "BAD JUDGMENT" TEST

Story A

1. T — that's what the story says.
2. ? — story doesn't say.
3. ? — tree, grass, other parts of truck *may* have been damaged but not necessarily.
4. T — that's what the story says.
5. ? — story says only that next-door neighbor was backing car but does not preclude this possibility.
6. F — story states the contrary.
7. T — that's what the story says.
8. ? — story doesn't say whether truck driver was a man.
9. ? — story does not preclude this possibility.

Story B

1. ? — Betty is not necessarily John's wife nor even a "Mrs." — she could be John's sister.
2. ? — story does not say that he did.
3. ? — story doesn't say — it could be that John or Betty left them scattered on retiring.
4. F — story states the contrary.
5. ? — story doesn't say.
6. F — story states the contrary.
7. ? — story doesn't say.
8. ? — story doesn't say that Betty Smith was a Mrs.
9. ? — story doesn't say what Smith thought of first.
10. ? — story doesn't say that Betty Smith was a Mrs.
11. ? — garden could be in same direction as living room but not necessarily.
12. ? — story doesn't say whether or not he saw a burglar.

Appendix F
Corporate Goals

I.   Continue to maintain, expand and improve our corporate hospital leadership position in providing comprehensive quality health care services to the region.

General Objectives

    A.   Establish Nebraska Methodist Hospital as a "Tertiary" level hospital.

    B.   Construct a new tower for patient services and beds at the 84th street location.

    C.   Establish a formal on-going system for short and long range medical and management planning.

    D.   Expand management, systems, and services to other hospitals.

    E.   Encourage medical staff to expand their efforts to provide programs, and services to the region.

    F.   Develop the corporate organizational structure and provide for adequate manpower.

    G.   Strive to gain more visibility and recognition for achievements in providing health care service.

II.   Assure the continued financial viability of the Nebraska Methodist Hospital.

Reprinted with the permission of J. W. Estabrook, Administrator, the Nebraska Methodist Hospital, Omaha, Nebraska.

General Objectives

A.   Expand and develop sources of revenue other than normal hospital services.

B.   Encourage the medical staff to develop their referral patterns on a regional basis.

C.   Develop management, systems, and programs to increase employee productivity.

D.   Develop management, systems, and programs to improve cost containment and effectiveness.

E.   Develop an internal financial reporting system that will measure achievement in productivity and cost containment.

III.   Continue to provide and expand an environment for employees to experience involvement, pride, security, and self-fulfillment.

General Objectives

A.   Develop training, communications, reporting systems, and financial incentives to strengthen and improve middle management from the lead-man through the departmental director.

B.   Keep employees informed of the achievements of their department and of the hospital.

C.   Maintain a comprehensive wage, benefit, and personnel program that will encourage and reward productive employees and remove non-productive employees.

D.   Develop training programs for employees and management aimed at improving technical and managerial skills.

IV.   Provide sufficient and properly allocated resources to consumers of health care services in the region at a competitive price.

General Objectives

A.   Develop reasonable standards for all aspects of patient care and treatment that will properly meet the

needs of the patient and reflect favorably on the
"image" of the hospital.

B.   Identify, and evaluate new services, in conjunction
with corporate planning activities, quantifying
manpower, equipment, and supplies, necessary to
develop the service.

C.   Monitor and improve all aspects of patient
scheduling from admission, through the
coordination of technical services, to dismissal.

D.   Evaluate present patient services and programs to
determine whether they should be maintained,
expanded, improved, diminished, or discontinued
in relationship to the needs of the community,
the needs of the medical staff, and the resource
of the hospital.

V.   Provide sufficient and properly allocated resources committed to
quality health education for the governing board, physicians,
students, employees, patients and the public.

General Objectives

A.   Continue to develop the School of Nursing and
other formal educational programs in order to
meet the needs of the hospital and the region.

B.   Develop a comprehensive program to provide
continuing education to employees throughout
the organization with emphasis toward technical
and managerial education.

C.   Provide for improved programs and methods to
inform and educate the governing board, medical
staff, and house officers and medical students
affiliated with the hospital.

D.   Continue to expand and improve patient education
and the health education of the public in
coordination with the medical staff.

VI.   Develop strategies designed to preserve the high quality private
practice of medicine and high quality hospital services in the
face of increasing social and governmental interference and
regulation.

General Objectives

A. Continue to monitor governmental activities and develop methods to communicate these to the governing board, medical staff, and management of the hospital.

B. Develop a mechanism to maximize the corporation ability to influence legislation.

C. Provide leadership in forming associations or affiliations with individuals or groups external to the hospital to communicate and develop strategies for countering undesirable regulation or interference.

D. Develop programs to react or to adjust to new or impending regulation.

Appendix G

Performance Descriptions— Nursing Department

TITLE: <u>Coordinator of Systems and Planning</u>

Department: Nursing Service

Responsible to: Director of Nursing

Definition: The Coordinator of Systems and Planning is a qualified professional nurse who is responsible for developing and implementing systems and procedures that will benefit patient care, personnel who perform them and promote cost effectiveness.

Performance Responsibilities	**Performance is Satisfactory When:**
A. <u>TO PATIENT</u>:	
1. Evaluate and develop nursing procedures affecting direct patient care for their effectiveness and safety.	1. Procedures are reviewed on a periodic basis. Ineffective procedures are identified and revised as needed.
2. Evaluate nursing care related to ancillary department procedures and assist with recommendations, revisions and clarifications.	2. Ancillary department procedures related to nursing care are reviewed periodically. Nursing care aspects are clarified and communicated to appropriate persons for revision.

Performance Responsibilities	Performance is Satisfactory When:
3. Minimize the cost of delivering quality patient care through the evaluation of systems for safety, quality and therapeutic considerations.	3. Demonstrable savings are recorded and verified. Such results are communicated to appropriate departmental and administrative personnel.
4. Implement change in procedures, policies and/or equipment effectively.	4. Appropriate personnel are informed of changes prior to their implementation.
5. Evaluations of products are conducted in a systematic manner.	5. Product evaluations include product demonstration for staff on trial units, written evaluations and summary of results which is presented to appropriate groups for consideration. Plans for appropriate inservicing for products are made.

B.   TO MEDICAL STAFF:

1. Assure that the systems and procedures for carrying out the patient care plans are safe and effective.	1. Recommendations from Medical Staff regarding specific systems or procedures are evaluated with appropriate actions taken.
2. Recommend and help to implement new systems and procedures which will contribute to more effective patient care programs.	2. New systems and procedures are presented to appropriate Medical Staff for review. Appropriate physicians are consulted in their development.

C.   TO DIRECTOR OF NURSING:

1. Suggest specific analytical studies of systems, methods, procedures and/or activities which offer significant potential for improvement.	1. Documentation of such recommendations and follow-up exists.
2. Submit monthly reports itemizing status of current projects and future projects to be undertaken.	2. Monthly reports are submitted within 7 days after the end of each month.

Performance Responsibilities	**Performance is Satisfactory When:**
3. Represent the Director of Nursing in contacts with other hospital departments on matters related to systems and procedures.	3. Such contacts are carried out skillfully so that cooperation is secured. The Director is requested to aid in such contacts when judgment so dictates.
4. Inform the Director at once of matters which she needs to know.	4. There is never an oversight in following the dictum "Never let your boss be surprised."
5. Assist Nursing personnel in implementing Nursing Unit objectives.	5. Assistance is rendered to nursing personnel in accordance with current priorities.
6. Develop an annual action program with objective to be accomplished by Systems and Planning.	6. Objectives are submitted prior to beginning of each fiscal year.

D.   TO OTHER DEPARTMENTS:

1. Assist other departments in improving methods, systems and/or procedures that may affect patient care directly and/or indirectly.	1. Interdepartmental contacts are made promptly when problems arise affecting patient care.
2. Provide special services if approved.	2. Cooperation rendered to other departments upon request.

E.   TO SELF:

1. Maintain an up-to-date knowledge and practice of nursing trends and new developments in the health field.	1. Participate in professional and clinical meetings pertinent to areas of special interest. Recommend, implement and/or share new knowledge and trends which effect and/or enhance patient care.
2. Continue to improve own skills in methods and procedures analysis, systems engineering, and business planning.	2. Achieve a sense of growth and increasing satisfaction in Systems and Planning accomplishments.

Performance Responsibilities	Performance is Satisfactory When:
3. Visit other local hospitals and business organizations with a reputation for success in improving problems similar to those being faced here.	3. Results of visits can be directly applied to current projects or to those planned for next year.
4. Become familiar with outside resources and services which can be utilized to help achieve objectives.	4. Resources contribute to cost effectiveness and achievement of objectives.

F.   <u>TO COMMITTEES</u>:

1. Participate on appropriate committees as member and/or resource person.	1. Committee membership responsibilities are accepted. Committee objectives are met.
2. Keep Systems and Planning committee informed of projects needing their consideration (ex. equipment, procedures, etc.)	2. Systems and Planning committee have opportunity to review projects and to make recommendations.

<u>QUALIFICATIONS</u>:

1. Graduate of an accredited School of Nursing.

2. Satisfactory references (personal and professional).

3. Current state licensure.

4. Advanced preparation in supervision, management, and research.

5. Demonstrate skills in establishing interpersonal and interdepartmental relationships.

6. Demonstrate working knowledge of hospital operation.

COMMUNITY GENERAL HOSPITAL

TITLE: Head Nurse

Department: Nursing Service

Supervises: RN, LPN, Nursing Assistant, Orderly, Ward Secretary,
Technicians and Unit Service Aides.

Purpose: Coordinate management and clinical activities on a
patient unit so that optimum quality of patient care
is delivered at minimum cost.

Performance Responsibilities	**Performance is Satisfactory When:**
A. TO PATIENTS:	
1. Plan safe, economical and efficient nursing care.	Relevant standards (i.e.) JCAH, ANA, NLN, governmental agencies) are met; and costs are controlled.
2. Plan and assist in patient teaching.	Patient demonstrates comprehension and performs satisfactorily.
3. See that quality patient care is given to each patient in accordance with quality standards.	Documentation on care plans and records, together with feedback, indicate that standards are met.
4. Give direct patient care as required.	Individual patient care needs are met, as in #3.
5. Formulate and utilize patient care plan to assist in resolving patient problems.	Documentation on the care plan indicates action on problems and progress toward discharge.
6. Act as liaison between patient, physician and family.	Patient and family understand and carry out physician's directions; feedback is provided to the physician.
B. TO MEDICAL STAFF:	
1. See that physician's orders are carried out.	Orders are carried out promptly and accurately.
2. Act as liasion between physician and patient care team.	Communications are clear, as documented and used on patient care plan.

Performance Responsibilities	Performance is Satisfactory When:
3. Question physician when communication is not clear.	No documented errors; no negative feedback.

C.   TO OWN NURSE MANAGER:

Performance Responsibilities	Performance is Satisfactory When:
1. Share appropriate communications with unit personnel.	Such communications are utilized and understood.
2. Assure adequate staffing.	Personnel are assigned for adequate coverage and optimum utilization.
3. Keep own nurse manager informed of unit activity, personnel problems and patients' conditions.	Appropriate information is communicated to own nurse manager.
4. Make out patient care assignments.	Assignments are made based upon competency of available personnel to meet patient care needs.
5. Seek assistance from nurse manager as necessary in solving clinical and management problems.	Specific instances of seeking and using such help occur.
6. Help with budget planning; operate unit within budget.	Budget is realistically related to patient care programs; and costs are within budget.

D. TO DEPARTMENT PERSONNEL:

Performance Responsibilities	Performance is Satisfactory When:
1. Act as leader, model, and innovator.	An example is set by using conferences, demonstrations, available resources, and the problem-solving method.
2. Delegate responsibilities within scope of personnel abilities.	Personnel and patients' needs are met.
3. Hold regular unit personnel meetings.	Active participation is evident and there is a feeling of satisfaction with unit meetings.
4. Promote an environment in which the patient care team can work cooperatively toward objectives.	Cooperative relationship exists among members of unit team.
5. Provide an opportunity for personnel staff development.	There is evidence of participation in continuing education activities.

Performance Responsibilities	Performance is Satisfactory When:
6. Assist staff with development and usage of nursing care plans.	Every patient care plan is current on a daily basis.
7. Counsel personnel when necessary.	Counseling is used for problem solving.

E. TO COMMITTEES:

1. Participate actively in selected committee activities.	Committee objectives are met.

F. TO OTHER DEPARTMENT PERSONNEL:

1. Aim for intra-departmental cooperation.	Good working relationship exists.
2. Keep open communication contact as needed to plan patient care.	Cooperation between departments exists and such cooperation favorably affects patient care.

G. TO OTHER ORGANIZATIONS:

1. Current membership in appropriate professional organization.	Participation proves satisfying and productive.

H. TO SELF:

1. Maintain sense of personal satisfaction; keep skills up to date.	Personal goals are met as related to job performance.
2. Participate in continuing education programs.	New learnings provide sense of growth and competency.

QUALIFICATIONS:

1. Graduate of Accredited School of Nursing; current state license.
2. Satisfactory performance in top staff nurse classification for a minimum of one year.
3. Demonstrated competence in management and leadership skills.
4. Successful completion of a management program for head nurses.

Appendix H
Cumberland County Health Department
Sample Forms

<hr>

Exhibit A

Maternal Child Health Interagency Report

CUMBERLAND COUNTY HEALTH DEPARTMENT

FAYETTEVILLE, NORTH CAROLINA

Follow-up: CFVH Room No. _______

( ) Emergency

( ) 1-2 Weeks   Clinic No. ____________

( ) 3-4 Weeks

Name ____ Race W ( ) NW ( )
HEAD OF FAMILY UNIT

Name _____________________________________ Relationship ____________
HEAD OF HOUSEHOLD UNIT PATIENT LIVES WITH

Address _____________________________________ Telephone ____________

Previous Address (If changed) ____

Financial Resource: ( ) Medically Indigent ( ) Medicaid ( ) DDS ( ) Military ( ) Private Doctor

Educational Level ____

Mother's Name _____________________	Infant's Name _______________ Sex M F
Maiden Name ______________________	DOB: _______ Time: _______ Dr._______
Age ____________ Marital Status M S W D Sep.	Birth: ( ) Single ( ) Twin No. 1 ( ) Twin No. 2
Date of Cl. Adm. __________ No. Visits ________	( ) Stillborn ( ) Abortion ( ) Neonatal death
Obstetrical history: Gravida ________ Para ______	Birth wt. ____________ Discharge wt. ____________
_______________________________________	Measurements: Length ______ Head ______ Chest ______
_______________________________________	Physical Exam: ( ) Normal APGAR ____________
STS ______________ RH ____________	_______________________________________
Delivered by: Dr. _________________________	_______________________________________
Week of gestation _________________________	_______________________________________
Labor & Delivery: Length ___________________	_______________________________________
Episiotomy __________ Laceration __________	Circumcision: Yes ____________ No ____________
Complications: _________________________	Discharge: Date ____________
_______________________________________	Feeding: ( ) Breast ( ) Formula ____________
_______________________________________	Problems: (Specify) ____________
Anesthesia: _____________________________	
Surgery: (Specify) _______________________	
_______________________________________	Plan for Medical Supervision:
Discharge date: _________________________	Nurse Screening Clinic: Appt. Requested ________
BP / Breast __________________	Date of Appt. ____________
Lochia _________________________________	Other: (Specify) ____________
Other: (Specify) _________________________	Date Referred to PHN ____________
Classes Attended: ( ) P. P./F.P.l. ( ) Baby Care	Signed: ____________________, R. N.
Date Referred to Clinic ___________________	RETURN ORIGINAL COPY TO CLINIC PRIOR TO APPOINTMENT CARBON COPY RETAINED BY DISTRICT PHN

<hr>

We thank the Cumberland County Health Department for their
permission to use the information and exhibits presented herewith.

Mother's Name ____

Notes by MCH Coordinating Nurse _______________________________

____

Notes by District PHN ____

____

Signed ___________________________________, R.N.

MCH REV. 4/72

Exhibit B

CUMBERLAND COUNTY HEALTH DEPARTMENT
Fayetteville, North Carolina

Nursing Standards for First Post Partum Home Visit

CONDITION	STANDARD	NURSE'S ACTION
I. Mother-Physical Assessment Objective:	To determine health status of mother, promote awareness of health state and provide nursing intervention as needed on first home visit two to four weeks post partum.	
A. Normal Breasts 1. Non-lactating	Dry, soft, nipples non-irritated, firm support bra.	Support present care routine
2. Lactating	Good quantity milk, firm nipples, erect and non-irritated, breasts rotated, adequate support bra.	Support present care routine.
B. B/P	Within range of 100/60 to 120/80 (?)	Check BP and record
C. Elimination 1. Bladder	No urgency or frequency, good bladder control, painfree emptying	Reinforce mother's knowledge of bladder function.
2. Bowels	Pre-pregnancy patterns resumed	Reinforce mother's knowledge of bowel function.
D. Involutional Process 1. Lochia	Absent to scanty amount, color brownish to white, free of odor.	Teach patient re: normal involutional lochia
2. Epsiotomy	Healing, non-painful	Support present routine
3. Abdomen	Non-painful, free of cramping (except during breast feeding)	Patient teaching Re: Fundus check
4. B.C. Method	Knowledge of two acceptable methods	If necessary PHN discuss each
5. Patient teaching	Prevention of perineal infection, intercourse frequency, p.p. physiological changes, P.P. clinic appointment.	If necessary PHN discusses each
E. Nutrition	Review basic diet and iron rich diet	Modify for individual patient Refer to P.P. diet standards
Γ. Physical Activities	Begin to resume normal daily activities, use P.P. exercises, and adequate rest.	Discuss progressive resumption and types of P.P. exercises, and rest needs.

CONDITION	STANDARD	NURSE'S ACTION
II. Infant-Physical Assessment Objective: To determine health status of infant, promote awareness of health state and provide nursing intervention as needed on first home visit, two to four weeks after birth.		
A. Skin	Clean and Clear (free of rash)	Reinforce skin care. Observe & record size & location of birth marks and/or mongolian spots.
B. Head	Normal shape & size in relation to other body proportions. Ant. fontanel open, flat. Post fontanel closed (or small opening) & flat.	Condition recorded Size recorded Size recorded
C. Scalp (hair area)	Clean, washed at least every other day.	Reinforce scalp cleansing
D. Ears	Top surface in line with external corner of eye, and symmetrical. Clean and normal in shape.	Reinforce bathing instructions including behind and in ears. (No Q-tips to be used.)
E. Eyes	Clear, clean and tearing	Reinforce correct cleansing
F. Nose	Both nostrils patent and free of discharge.	Reinforce care
G. Mouth & Throat	Mucosa clear and palate closed	Reinforce oral care including water offered following formula to reduce milk coating and luke warm temperature of formula.
H. Neck	Supple, free of masses and irritation.	Reinforce cleansing instructions including folds of neck.
I. Chest	Non-retracting respirations Breasts non-enlarged	Condition recorded
J. Abdomen	Soft, and no palpable masses	Condition recorded
K. Umbilical Cord	On and dry, off and healing. Abscence of herniation.	Reinforce umbilical care.
L. Genitalia 1. Female	Vaginal os patent, folds non-swollen, area clean and free of irritation.	Reinforce vaginal care.
2. Male	Testicles descended and scrotal sac non-swollen. Circumsized penis healed, clean and foreskin easily retractible	Reinforce continued observance of sac for swelling and record. Record position of testicles. Reinforce retraction of foreskin.
	Uncircumsized penis clean and able to visualize meatus	Reinforce retraction of foreskin.

CONDITION	STANDARD	NURSE'S ACTION
M. Extremities		
1. Upper	Simultaneous movement and full ROM. Hands-normal appearance, shape, and size.	Record findings
2. Lower	Hips-bilateral full ROM Legs-straight and equal with symmetrical posterior folds. Feet-straight	Record findings
N. Spinal Column	Straight, spinal process palpable and free of masses and/or sinuses	Record condition
O. Bowel	Anal os patent, free of tags and irritation. Stools—color, consistency and frequency relate adequately to type of formula intake.	Reinforce mother's daily observance of bowel habits and knowledge of themometer use.
P. Bladder	Voids every ½ hour, stream continuous not intermittant, urine stains yellow and has ammonia-like odor.	Reinforce frequent diaper changes and genital cleansing. Thorough diaper washing methods.
Q. Reflexes	Infant demonstrates grasp, startle, sucking and head turning (fencing) reflexes	Record findings
R. Nutrition		
1. Formula	Identify formula brand, 24 hour quantity, and frequency of feedings. Identify preparation method of choice to patient.	Modify for individual patient (Refer to infant formula procedure.) Review method chosen. (Aseptic, terminal)
2. Solids	Identify type of solids and frequency, if already introduced	Discuss introduction and progression of solids. (Refer to infant feeding procedure)
S. Safety	See Section IV Environment	

III. Environment
   Objective: Evaluate physical and emotional environment and determine mode of child care.

CONDITION	STANDARD	NURSE'S ACTION

A. Physical (Dwelling)	Adequate water source
	  1. Clean well water and pump
	  2. Indoor plumbing
	Adequate heating and cooking source. Screens on windows and doors.
		Record Findings

B. Emotional	Mother holds child securely, with ease, and relates to child. Family accepts child. Father supports family emotionally and financially.	Record observations Reinforce

CONDITION	STANDARD	NURSE'S ACTION
C. Child Care	Adequate care given	Determine and record who gives care and where
D. Safety	Measures appropriate for age	Record and reinforce

IV. Equipment
   Objective: Determine number of care items and inform mother of additional items needed.

A. Mother	Firm support bra & sanitary pads	Record findings Reinforce usage
B. Baby 1. Clothing	Diapers-24 cloth and/or pampers, tops-6 Receiving blankets-2	Record findings Reinforce usage
2. Hygiene	Soap-ivory, dial, Safeguard personal towel	Record findings Reinforce usage
3. Formula	6 bottles, nipples and caps (formula and water) Can Opener Refrigeration Formula container and cover	Record findings Reinforce usage
4. Foods	Personal spoon and dish Solids appropriate for age level	Record findings Reinforce usage
5. Sleeping	Separate bed with firm pad or mattress. Bed linens-crib sheets, puddle pads, mats or plastic pads, blanket	Record findings Reinforce usage

Exhibit C

RETROSPECTIVE AUDIT SHEET

<u>First Post-Partum Home Visit</u>

Patient's Name ________________________

```
         CODE:   YES = Present
                 NO  = Not present         Date of Home Visit ________________
                 NA  = Not assessible
                 V   = Variation           YES    NO    NA    V     Comments
```

I. Mother

    A. Breasts   96%*
       1. Condition of non-lactating breasts
       2. Condition of lactating breasts

    B. Recording of BP findings   100%

    C. Elimination   96%
       1. Bladder elim. noted
       2. Bladder control noted
       3. Bowel pattern noted

    D. Vagina   90%
       1. Description of lochia
       2. Condition of epsiotomy
       3. Perineal self care noted
       4. Perineal teaching including:
          a. hygiene
          b. intercourse frequency
          c. family planning
          d. next clinic visit

    E. Diet and exercise   100%
       1. Teaching re diet noted
       2. Teaching re PP exercises noted

II. Infant

    A. Skin condition noted   96%

    B. Head notations re: condition of:
       1. Shape   96%
       2. Size   96%
       3. Size of Ant. Fontanel   96%
       4. Size of Post. Fontanel   96%
       5. Eyes   96%
       6. Ears   96%
       7. Nose   96%
       8. Mouth/Throat   96%

    C. Condition of neck   96%

    D. Chest   96%
       1. Condition of respirations
       2. Condition of breasts

    E. Abdomen   90%
       1. Condition of tone
       2. Condition of cord

      * See text for explanation of %.

First Post-Partum Home Visit

Patient's Name ___________________________

Date of Home Visit ___________________________

Audit Sheet		YES	NO	NA	V	Comments
II. F. Genitalia	96%					
1. Female-appearance normal os patient						
2. Male-circumcised & condition	96%					
uncircumcised & foreskin retractibility testicles & scrotal sac app. normal	96%					
G. Extremities						
1. Upper movement noted	96%					
2. Lower movement noted	96%					
position noted	96%					
H. Spinal position noted	96%					
I. Bowel						
condition of anal os	96%					
bowel activity noted	100%					
taught use of thermometer	50%					
J. Bladder						
diaper condition when changed	96%					
K. Remaining primary reflexes noted	96%					
L. Diet	100%					
1. Formula type noted Quantity of intake						
2. Type solids noted Teaching re progression noted Freq. of feedings noted						
M. Teaching re safety noted	96%					
III. Child Care	100%					
A. Who gives noted						
B. Where care given noted						
IV. Equipment						
A. Mother during 1st 2 wks PP.	100%					
peri-care noted pads used noted						

First Post-Partum Home Visit   Patient's Name _______________________

                                            Date of Home Visit ___________________

Audit Sheet   YES   NO   NA   V   Comments

B. Baby
   1. Clothing items noted
   2. Hygiene items noted
   3. Formula items noted
   4. Solid food items noted
   5. Sleeping arrangement items
                    noted

V. Environment

   A. House
      1. Water source noted
      2. Heating source noted
      3. Window and door screens noted
      4. Cooking source noted

VI. Emotional Climate

   A. Mother's handling of child
   B. Mother's relationship with child
   C. Family acceptance of child
   D. Type of support from father

Exhibit D

QUALITY CONTROL CHECK: PUBLIC HEALTH NURSING AUDIT

Data must be held in STRICT confidence and MUST NOT BE FILED with patient's record.

All entries to be complete by trained clerk.

1. Name of Patient: 2. Sex: 4. Admission date:
                                                      type:

(Last)   (First)   3. Age: 5. Discharge date:

6. Nursing Agency: 7. Number of visits to patient by agency:

8. Complete diagnosis(es):

9. Was patient hospitalized immediately   10. Medical supervision:
   prior to PHN service:

Yes No. Days No Unknown   N/A   Private Ward   OPD/Cl.   N/A
 □   □   □   □   □   □   □   □   □

11. Patient referred to PHN by:
    Hospital   Hospital   Patient's   MCH   Other
    Nurse   Social Worker   M.D.   Family   Nurse   Specify: N/A   Unknown
      □   □   □   □   □   □   □   □

12. Patient discharged from PHN to:
    Self-   Family   Rehospit-   Other PHN   Not Dis-   Other
    Care   Care   alized   Died   Agency   charged   Specify: Unknown
      □   □   □   □   □   □   □   □

13. All nursing entries signed by   14. Nursing entries show whether made by
    name and dated: public health, professional, practical,
                                              student nurse, physiotherapist, other:
    YES   NO   YES   NO
     □   □   □   □

15. Plan of care is recorded: YES   NO
                                    □   □

	YES	NO
16. Were there any accidents or special incidents?	___	___
a. If yes, chart indicates report was submitted to administration	___	___
b. Or, report is part of the chart	___	___
17. Nursing admission entry shows assessment of patient's condition:		
physical	___	___
emotional	___	___
18. Nursing discharge entry shows assessment of patient's condition:		
phsical	___	___
emotional	___	___

EXPLANATION OF EXHIBITS

Exhibit A: The Interagency Report Form

The maternal child health interagency report is initiated by the maternal and child health nurse working in the hospital who completes Section 1 (as well as the top of Section 2). Section 1 serves as the data base on mother and infant for the district public health nurse who makes the first postpartum visit to the mother and infant.

Section 2 of the maternal child health interagency report serves as the progress notes and plan of care for mother and infant. The lower half is completed by the district public health nurse after the initial visit to mother and infant.

Exhibit B: Standards for First Postpartum Visit

Qualitative standards were established for the physical assessment and care of both mother and infant and for child care, equipment necessary for care in the home, the physical environment of the home, and the emotional climate in the home.

Exhibit C: Retrospective Audit for First Postpartum Visit

The same standard (Exhibit B) serves also as the basis for the retrospective audit for the audit topic: First postpartum home visit. A Retrospective Audit Sheet was designed to retrieve the necessary data (Exhibit C). The percentages on this form indicate 96% or below as acceptable for many elements. A 100% standard for data gathering on home visits is felt by the district public health nurses to be unrealistic due to occasional presence of neighbors and friends. Every effort is made by the nurse to avoid embarrassing the mother or family members.

Exhibit D: Quality Control Check of First Postpartum Visit

An audit of the nursing process is carried out for the same mother and infant. A quality control check form, Exhibit D, is used for this purpose. It is adapted from the form provided by Maria C. Phaneuf in The Nursing Audit.[1]

Notes

1. Maria C. Phaneuf, The Nursing Audit: Profile for Excellence (New York: Appleton-Century-Crofts, 1972), p. 22.

Appendix I

Maslow's Theory of Human Motivation

Abraham Maslow

Abraham Maslow was born April 1, 1908, in a slum district of Brooklyn, New York. His early years of schooling were spent in New York city schools. His college years were spent at City College of New York, then Cornell, and later Wisconsin, where his interests turned to psychology. He was a shy, studious, brilliant student . . . an achiever, following his own learning inclinations. After graduation, he worked for E.L. Thorndike, the Watsonian disciple (and developer of intelligence tests) at Teacher's College, Columbia University. Later he taught for fourteen years at Brooklyn College—until he moved to Brandeis University near Boston, Massachusetts. During his Brooklyn years he was able to learn much from his contacts with Max Wertheimer (the founding member of the gestalt school), Erich Fromm, Karen Horney, Kurt Goldstein, Ruth Benedict (the renowned anthropologist) and Alfred Adler.

In the early thirties, after studying human learning, he concluded that success and reward has a far more powerful effect than failure or punishment. Later, he became disenchanted with the kind of clinical psychology that was based upon the study of abnormal personalities—of sick people. So he decided to study the healthiest people he could find—the most creative, productive, happiest human beings. The result made history.

Maslow's findings are widely published, interpreted and used throughout the world. He presented the need hierarchy and its relations to motivation in his now-classic book, *Motivation and Personality*. Though widely acclaimed by many, it met with skepticism from a wide spectrum of the traditional psychologists. Maslow was seen as a renegade and was virtually ostracized by the American Psychological Association. Later, however, in the midsixties, he was elected to the presidency of APA.

He became a founder of the Association for Humanistic Psychology and the recognized leader of "The Third Force"—the name he gave to the serious and fast-growing movement he fathered that challenged the most basic precepts on which the study of man had been based for a century. It challenged Freud's dictatorship of the subconscious and the mechanistic world of the behaviorists. In their stead, it proposed a new philosophy of man, an optimistic human awareness that sets man free to be man, to create and grow, to control his choices and goals.

Maslow died of a second heart attack, in California, in June 1970. He lives on in the hearts, minds, and work of a great host of mankind whose lives he touched in so many ways. He remains a force for good in a world coping with so many forms of the bad.

Henry Geiger, who wrote the introduction to the Maslow book, *The Farther Reaches of Human Nature* explains the deserved popularity of Maslow's works.

> *People who read him understand why. He has a*
> *psychology that applies to them . . . . All through his*
> *work one finds exposed nodes open to intuitive*
> *verification, good enough for any man of hungry*
> *common sense. These "insights" make people keep*
> *on reading Maslow. . . . Nearly all his writing gives*
> *off sparks.*

Exhibit A

MASLOW'S THEORY OF HUMAN MOTIVATION

The Hierarchy of Needs

The human being is motivated by a number of basic needs. It is the
unsatisfied needs which have the greatest influence on behavior. Once a need
has been gratified it has little effect on motivation. A want that is satisfied
is no longer a want. The first two needs are basic needs, the latter three are
growth needs.

1.   Survival (Physiological) needs represent our needs for food, clothing,
      shelter, and other things which are essential to our existence. So long
      as these needs go unsatisfied, the individual is little concerned with other
      needs and his efforts will be directed toward satisfaction in this area.

2.   Security (Safety) needs. Once the individual's survival needs are satisfied
      to at least a minimum degree, his dominant needs become security needs.
      His efforts are directed toward satisfaction in this area. Security needs
      include physical safety, job tenure, insurance, pensions, etc.

3.   Social, (Love, affection, belonging) needs. When the individual has
      minimum satisfaction of his survival and security needs, belongingness
      needs become important to him. These are the needs for love, acceptance,
      and approval by others—his family, his friends, those with whom he
      works.

4.   Status (Esteem, self-worth) needs. The individual whose survival,
      security and belongingness needs are satisfied in at least a minimum
      fashion then becomes concerned with esteem needs—the need for recog-
      nition and status. Whereas belongingness needs are more or less passive,
      esteem needs involve the active favorable reactions of others. The esteem
      need also includes the individual's need for self-respect, or self-esteem.

5.   Self-Actualizing (Self-Fulfillment) needs. If the survival, security, and
      belongingness and esteem needs are all satisfied to at least a minimum
      degree, the individual's dominant need becomes self-fulfillment. This
      need is the individual's desire to become his best self, to realize his
      capabilities to the fullest, to know that he is making his greatest
      contribution to humanity.

Adapted from *Motivation and Personality* by A. H. Maslow, 2nd Edition,
Harper & Row, New York, 1970; and *The Third Force* (The Psychology of
Abraham Maslow) by Frank Goble, Pocket Books, New York City, 1971.
Reprinted by permission of Harper & Row Publishers, Inc. 1970.

Exhibit B

UNDERSTANDING MOTIVATION

Why I Do What I Do

I HAVE FIVE HUMAN NEEDS. I DO WHAT I DO BECAUSE I MUST SATISFY MY NEEDS.

To Survive

I need to get food, shelter, air; things I need to stay alive.

To Feel Secure

I need to feel secure at home, on my job, in my life situation . . .
within myself.

For Meaningful Social Contacts

I need such contacts to give me a sense of belonging, to share
love and affection, to know I am wanted.

For Status

I need a sense of self-esteem, the respect of others, pride in
my ability and accomplishments, a sense of self-worth.

For Self-Actualization

I need to continue growing toward becoming my best possible
self and greater self-realization.

Beyond these needs I have *metaneeds*, the search for the "being values" ("B"
for short), the ultimate values which are intrinsic. I need meaning in my life,
to worship, to satisfy the human values of being including truth, beauty,
goodness, simplicity, wholeness, and others.

Exhibits B and C are adapted from A. H. Maslow, *Motivation and Personality*,
2nd Ed. (New York: Harper & Row, 1970); idem, *The Farther Reaches of
Human Nature* (New York: The Viking Press, 1971); idem, *Toward a
Psychology of Being* (New York: Van Nostrand Reinhold, 1968). For more
information on metaneeds idem, *Religions, Values, and Peak Experiences*
(New York: The Viking Press, 1970).

Exhibit C
WHY MY NEEDS ARE NEVER FULLY SATISFIED

Why My Needs Are Never Fully Satisfied

*I CAN UNDERSTAND MYSELF AND OTHERS BETTER WHEN I RECOGNIZE
THE RELATIONSHIP BETWEEN MY NEEDS AND MY MOTIVATION.*

> If my survival is threatened, other needs become less
> important. I do what I must do to stay alive.
>
> When I know I will survive, my need for security and safety
> becomes important. I act in ways which I think will help me to
> reach at least a minimum level of security.
>
> Then, with survival and security needs satisfied to some
> degree, I begin to seek more social satisfactions (belonging
> to a group; giving and receiving affection).
>
> I seek also more of a sense of status, esteem, and self-worth.
> And I reach out for greater self-actualization and personal
> growth.
>
> Having attained a sense of satisfaction for all of the
> foregoing, I still want more. I strive for a higher level
> of aliveness, uniqueness, justice, order, perfection,
> self-sufficiency, playfulness, richness, effortlessness,
> and the other "B" values—the metaneeds.

I behave this way because I am a human being with human needs that must
be satisfied. Other people are like me, all striving to satisfy their needs too.
That's why we act the way we do.

If I can't meet the need that I feel most, then I hurt. When I satisfy a need,
I feel good—but immediately another need takes its place. When I satisfy
a need it is no longer a motivator for me, but another need is.

I am motivated when I feel desire or want or yearning or wish or lack.

Glossary

Agency: A business or service acting for others; a hospital, nursing home, mental health center, public health department, or other healthcare organization.

Annual Budgetary Planning (ABP): An organized approach to program planning for quality patient care with cost containment through decentralized nursing responsibility for budget preparation and control.

Apperceptive Mass: The associational area of your brain; what you have to react with.

Authority: The sanction to act within a prescribed area of responsibility.

Budget: An itemized summary of probable expenses and income for a given period.

Clinical Track: Career development and promotion via specialized clinical positions as contrasted with nursing management and administration.

Concept: An idea; a theory; a general understanding, thought, or notion that grows out of specific instances or occurrences.

Conceptualize: To form ideas, concepts, or theories; to perceive the broad, integrative relationships of diverse elements.

Controlling: Evaluating, measuring, and feedback function; the link between Doing and Planning in the management process.

Diagram: A schematic or plan; a graphic representation of relationships between parts of a whole.

Doing: The implementation phase of the management process; carrying out the plans.

Element: A fundamental, essential, or irreducible constituent of a composite entity.

Function: Assigned duty or activity; specific occupation or role; thus the *management functions* are planning, doing, and controlling—the three cyclical components of the management process.

Goal: A specific statement of purpose; aim.

Head Nurse: The nurse manager with 24-hour (or day shift only) responsibility on a single patient care unit for clinical nursing care, patient teaching, staff development, and unit management.

Healthcare: The process of maintaining optimal functioning of an organism with freedom from disease and abnormality; as an adjective, descriptive of those persons or agencies devoted to assisting others in maintaining or returning to a normal, healthy condition.

Human Mode: Those aspects of management, nursing, and patient care that focus on the motivation and behavior of the patients and the nursing staff, emphasizing the interpersonal skills in nursing.

Job Enrichment: Structuring jobs so they are more satisfying to employees.

Leadership: The skills used in persuading others to do what has to be done and in convincing them that they want to do it.

Major Job Segments: The responsibilities and duties required of a nursing employee to get the work done and meet objectives.

Management: The process of getting the right things done at the right time through and with the right people.

Management by Objectives (MBO): A results-oriented philosophy and system of managing, using mutually established objectives, target dates, and evaluation of performance. (See also **Nursing by Objectives.**)

Management Track: Career development and promotion via nursing administration and nurse manager roles as contrasted with the clinically oriented promotional opportunities.

Matrix Organization: An organic, adaptive organization structure that provides for functional interdepartmental and interdisciplinary leadership to achieve common goals; graphically, this structure appears as a grid (matrix) with hierarchical (vertical) coordination through departmentalization and the formal chain of command as well as simultaneous lateral (horizontal) coordination across departments.

Model: The structural relationships among the elements of a concept or system; the framework within which an idea exists; a means of communicating a concept.

Motive Power: That element in the working relationship between two or more persons which determines whose plan of action is dominant; characterized by an ability to see the broad picture, a desire to change things, and a willingness to be measured by results.

Nurse Manager: A nurse whose regular job responsibility is the management of personnel (such as director of nursing service, patient care coordinator, supervisor, head nurse).

Nursing Audit: A method for assuring documentation of the quality of nursing care in keeping with the standards of the agency, the nursing department, and the professional, governmental, and accrediting groups.

Nursing by Objectives (NBO): A results-oriented philosophy and system of managing a department of nursing using mutually established objectives, target dates for completion, and evaluation of performance.

Nursing Care: Delivery of direct care to patients.

Nursing Process: The four cyclical steps of sizing up the patient's needs and problems *(assessing)*, deciding what to do *(planning)*, securing action *(implementing)*, and seeing if the action helped with the needs and problems *(evaluating)*.

Nursing Services: Delivery of direct care to patients plus those elements of nursing done on behalf of the patient but not necessarily in his presence.

Objective: A specific task-oriented statement of results to be achieved to accomplish a goal.

Objectives, Jointly Developed: Objectives mutually prepared by the nursing employee with the nurse manager of that person.

Organizational Development (OD): A process of creating a climate for organizational change and growth through the development and effective utilization of nursing personnel and other resources.

Patient Care Coordinator: The nurse manager who provides administrative leadership for two or more patient care units, with 24-hour responsibility for clinical nursing care, patient teaching, staff development, and unit management.

Performance Description: A statement of the *purpose* of a job, the major performance *responsibilities* (grouped by the persons *to whom* the responsibilities exist), and *measures* of satisfactory performance.

Performance Evaluation: The regular review an appraisal of personnel performance (see also **Results-Oriented Performance Evaluation—ROPEP**).

Philosophy: Those beliefs, principles, and values that serve as a basis for action and behavior.

Planning: Thinking ahead, determining what shall be done; the management process of establishing objectives, defining problems and opportunities, setting goals, and developing strategy and tactics for actions.

Primary Nurse: The RN who has been assigned a small case load of patients and who serves as the leader for the care of those patients from admission through discharge in a hospital setting in which primary nursing is the basic system of care.

Primary Nursing: An alternative method of patient care in hospitals with one RN assigned and accountable for a small case load of individual patients, permitting a one-to-one patient-nurse relationship (with the focus on the nursing process) and a problem-solving approach based on the patient's needs and problems.

Problem-Oriented Nursing System (PONS): A process for assessing, planning, implementing, and evaluating patient care based on identified principles of nursing practice; involving the systematic recording of each patient's data base and identified problems; with an initial plan of care, progress notes, and discharge planning keyed to the problem list; and supported by a nursing audit program within service and continuing education as relevant.

Professional: A person with the knowledge, skills, experience, confidence, flexibility, and performance results that lead to recognition for a line of work.

Program Performance Plan (PPP): A long range schedule of the interrelated steps required to effect a desired result, objective, or goal.

Quality Assurance Program (QAP): A planned approach to aid each healthcare agency meet patient care goals through compliance with the standards established by the accrediting agencies and professional groups.

Responsibility: A duty or activity a person is expected to perform; that for which a person is held accountable.

Results-Oriented Performance Evaluation Program (ROPEP): A method of establishing and implementing an evaluation plan for nursing personnel based on performance descriptions with measurable standards of quality and quantity.

Schedule: A timetable or production plan; in nursing management, it usually refers to the time sheets showing planned work days for personnel.

Scientific Management: A type of management based on measurement plus control; the term was selected by Frederick Winslow Taylor ("the father of scientific management") and his colleagues in the early years of the twentieth century.

Skill: Proficiency in a way of doing something using one's hands, body, and brain.

Standard: An acknowledged measure of comparison for quantitative or qualitative value; criterion, norm.

Standards of Care: Clearly defined measures of comfort, techniques, clinical observation, perception, interpretation, and judgments used in initiating nursing actions and evaluating therapeutic results.

Standards of Performance: Written statements that define and provide a measure of how well employees are expected to carry out their responsibilities and meet their objectives.

Standards of Service: Clearly defined measures for the planning and managing of nursing care, staffing the units, making work assignments, keeping records, implementing policies and procedures, and maintaining interpersonal relations.

System: A group of interrelated elements forming a collective entity.

Target Date: The date by which an objective is to be achieved.

Technical Mode: Those aspects of management, nursing, and patient care that are dependent largely on treatments, systems, and procedures of a technical nature.

Technique: A design for an action plan, procedure, or program to assist the nurse manager to perform one or more management functions.

Time Sheet: The planned personnel work schedule; and/or the record of days and hours worked.

Transactional Analysis in Problem Solving (TAPS): A model for effective problem solving and decision making based upon the study of ego states exhibited by human beings.

Wide-Track Careers in Nursing (WTC): A viable system for providing selective career options on both the clinical track and the management track, using agency-developed criteria for continuing education opportunities and the related qualifying procedures.

Index

About the Authors

Warren and Joan Ganong are a unique husband and wife healthcare management counseling team. As President and Vice-President of Ganong Healthcare Management Consultants, their consulting and facilitating work takes them into practically every area of the healthcare industry throughout the United States of America. Their clients include general hospitals and medical centers, state and county agencies and facilities, VA hospitals, mental health clinics, nursing homes, schools of nursing, and other educational centers.

Joan began her working career as a psychiatric aide, then became interested in nursing and received her diploma from St. Luke's Hospital School of Nursing, New York City. She studied at Hunter College for her B.S. in Education, and at the University of Maryland for her M.S. in Nursing. She has held positions at every job level in nursing service and nursing education in hospitals ranging from St. Luke's Hospital in New York City to Johns Hopkins Hospital and Union Memorial Hospital in Baltimore, Maryland, and Presbyterian-University Hospital in Pittsburgh, Pennsylvania. She is an Adjunct Assistant Professor in Continuing Education at the University of North Carolina School of Nursing in Chapel Hill. She serves also on the faculty of the University of Minnesota Independent Study Program in Patient Care Administration.

Warren's background is in industrial engineering, labor relations, and organizational development — with a quarter century of consulting experience for healthcare agencies. He acquired his B.S. in Industrial Engineering from Northeastern University, Boston, with graduate work at M.I.T. He is a certified management consultant and past president of the Association of Management Consultants, and Pittsburgh Management Consultants Association, and the Pittsburgh Chapter of the Society for Advancement of Management.

Both Joan and Warren teach extensively in university, technical institute, school, business, and on-the-job settings. In their consulting work the Ganongs place emphasis on helping the personnel of client organizations to help themselves. This involves staff development —

experiential training in newer methods, techniques, and skills. Known as "The People People," the Ganongs have written and illustrated the HELP Series of Management Guides as an aid to administrators, department heads, nurse managers and healthcare educators everywhere.